It's My Time: Planning a Holistic Retirement

Brian McNicol

Muthu Pannirselvam

A comprehensive guide to health, wealth, relationships and leisure in the best years of your life.

Disclaimer

The information contained in this book is given in good faith and has been derived from sources believed to be accurate at the time of writing. No liability will be accepted by the authors or publishers for actions taken by any person on the strength of this information alone. It is recommended that professional independent advice be sought.

Editor

Anthony Skinner

First published in July 2021 by Arthur Phillip Books

Cover designed by Brian McNicol and Muthu Pannirselvam

Dedication

To my wife, Annette, who has been by my side for over 45 years. She has inspired and supported me and I look forward to spending more time with her and enjoying many more adventures in the years to come.

To my children and grandchildren who provide me with so much joy and pride.

To my friends and acquaintances who have provided the inspiration for this book. Thank you.

Contents

Preparation for old age should begin not later than one's teens. A life which is empty of purpose until 65 will not suddenly become filled on retirement.

Arthur E. Morgan

You do not have to look too far to find advice on how people can plan financially for retirement. However, there is often an information gap on the psychological and health aspects of retirement and how it affects you, your partners and your marriage. It is important that people start thinking about what can be the most productive, or the most challenging, years of their lives. The choices made now may significantly impact on the 15, 20 or 30 years of your retirement.

This book is the first of two books we are writing on retirement and this one is designed to help you think about, and plan for, retirement. The second book, Retirementor, is essentially for those that have taken a step closer, or are retired, and relates the experiences and advice of people who have retired. Both retirees and people planning retirement will get benefits from both books.

Mention the word retirement to anybody and it will conjure up different visions and thoughts; from excitement to anxiety and trepidation for each person. These thoughts and visions are fluid and will change over time. Instead of the boundaries and structures imposed by work, retirement is a new chapter still to be written. Any boundaries, structure or expectations are those set by the individual.

We will look at a little history and the concept of retirement and ask the question "Is retirement dead?" Whether retirement is an outdated concept is debatable. What is undeniable is that we are entering uncharted waters. Never before has there been so many millions of people either entering or about to enter retirement. In the United States of America alone, it is estimated that there are about 77 million Baby Boomers about to enter retirement. In Australia, this figure is about 5 million. Governments across the world, for years, have known of this coming retiree tsunami but most have done little to prepare for it.

For people in their 20s and early 30s, retirement is in the distant future and not really a consideration. There are too many other things to occupy the mind – career, nights out with friends, travel and possibly a serious relationship or marriage.

Even in their late 30s, most people aren't thinking about retirement. Yes, they may be starting to get tired of working but marriage, starting a family, and setting up a house are the main focus.

In their 40s, people may start to think about how nice retirement would be but they are basically shackled to their job. They have a family to support, children to educate and therefore retirement is still a distant dream.

Depending upon when a person got shackled to their job, through family, children's education or the desire to climb the corporate ladder, those in their 50s might now start to recognise a variety of signals. Their body may be starting to slow down physically or advertisements for ocean cruises or over 55s living are now starting to be noticed whereas previously they attracted no attention.

In their late 50s and early 60s, reality hits for most people. There is a realisation that the retirement that they had longed for in earlier years was now almost upon them and many are not financially ready for it. Sometimes, there is the dreaded fear that retirement may come earlier than expected due to redundancies or business closure. That is why it is important to plan for retirement even if you have no intention of retiring. Do not put retirement planning into the too-hard basket. Planning for retirement involves much more than just money.

What are we going to do and will we be able to live comfortably for the next 20 or 30 years? Can we rely on a government pension?

Most people think that planning for retirement is all about our financial security. A large industry has grown up around providing financial advice to retirees and future retirees. There are other industries focusing on helping us to spend our retirement nest egg on overseas holidays, cruises to exotic destinations, or fitting out a new four-wheel drive vehicle and caravan to join the grey nomads driving around Australia.

The reality is that preparing for retirement and living in retirement is a lot more than planning for our financial future. Yes, having a secure financial future is important but, as we will learn in this book, it is only one small part of preparing for, and enjoying, our retirement. We also hope to answer a question that is often thought about and sometimes asked: 'how will I know when I am ready to leave work?' This question is often related to our financial status but, as we will see, it depends on other factors as well.

In the 1970s, I worked for a company where people could retire at 60. The company had a good superannuation scheme so money was seldom a problem for these retirees. Every couple of months an email would go out to workers advising of the death of a former colleague. This often happened within a couple of years of their retirement. The company then lowered the retirement age to 55 but the same trend continued. Financially, these retirees had no problems receiving a pension from a very good superannuation fund and possibly after 30 – 35 years of service. One of the common threads amongst the deceased retirees was a lack of social network. Their life revolved around work and they were dysfunctional without it. For some this was compounded by leaving their friends and families behind to start a new life in a warmer climate.

Those nearing retirement need to plan how they will spend their days otherwise they can lose the purpose and direction in their life. How do you keep mentally and physically active now? How do you connect socially and create new social networks? How may this need to change, if necessary, between now and retirement?

This book is partly based on personal experience, both historical and current. I left work in 2011 with little idea of planning for what I would do in retirement. Like most people, I had thought that retirement was all about money. My wife retired in October 2019. In hindsight, she was a lot better prepared than I was and with a far broader outlook on retirement than I had.

It is an exciting time for Baby Boomers. They are entering a new retirement, one that no other generations have faced. Medical science now gives us the opportunity to live longer, to live more productive lives, but these advances in medicine have created other challenges in what has previously been called retirement.

As we discuss in this book, to prepare for retirement and to enjoy a long and happy retirement requires planning. We need to plan not just for a few years but long-term, maybe the next 30 years. It has been said that people spend more time planning an overseas holiday or a road trip than they do planning for their retirement. Planning for a long, happy and fulfilling retirement is more like a marathon than a sprint race so we need to prepare. It is never too late (or early) to start planning for retirement. Retirement is an ongoing process; its impact is significant and long-lasting.

National Seniors Australia published a report in 2012 which had some interesting, but also disturbing, facts. When asked whether pre-retirees had a plan, only 62 per cent said they had some kind of financial plan, $24 - 27$ per cent had plans for their health and $17 - 26$ per cent had plans in place for lifestyle, social and community engagement in retirement. How many then have followed through on their plans?

Today, there is also a new reality to retirement. You now have to be more active and take retirement planning into your own hands. How your retirement will look is entirely up to you.

You are in a privileged position at this time in your lives. With a little knowledge, a little tenacity and time, you can do anything.

Whilst this book is about transitioning and planning for retirement, do not wait for retirement to enjoy the life you want.

The Boomers have always been rebels and that non-conforming streak will continue in retirement.

We have attempted to provide the knowledge; it is up to you to provide the tenacity and time so that you can fully enjoy growing old (dis)gracefully.

Retirement is wonderful if you have two essentials: much to live for, and much to live on. (Anonymous)

We would also like to add another two essentials: health and relationships.

Chapter 1

Retirement – is it an outdated concept?

Retirement at 65 is ridiculous. When I was 65, I still had pimples.

George Burns

What is retirement?

Many definitions of retirement would mention that a person:

- is leaving and formally withdrawing from their employment
- is permanently ceasing their job or profession
- has reached a certain age and is transitioning from a job to a lifestyle dominated by leisure
- is at the end of a particular social status resulting from a professional role.

Some people also identify retirement as the start of the fourth stage of life. This follows the three earlier stages of infancy, learning/education, and employment.

In the past, retirement was associated with reaching a certain age. A person finished their working life, had a few years to spend time with grandchildren, and go fishing or travel before they ultimately departed this life. In 1900, a man might have expected to spend less than two years in retirement. Others may have lived a little longer but not necessarily in the best of health. Since the Second World War, retirement was something that people always looked forward to. There was some type of retirement party to send the retiree off to enjoy those short years. Work back then often involved a large amount of regimentation and, in part, boredom. There was also a sense of entitlement to the pension, having paid taxes for all those working years. Even though the retirement years may have been short, they were regarded as the golden years and had a positive connotation for most people.

Better health care and nutrition has seen life expectancy in retirement increase by about 18 years in 2000 and it is expected to increase further in the coming years. For most retirees today, that concept of retirement is dead. Today, retirement has taken on a whole new meaning for most people. It is a time of new opportunities, a time to do things that you did not have time for due to work and family commitments. It is a time to be the 'real you' without the constraints of what is expected of you, by your work or profession.

There is also some debate about words that have been traditionally related to retirement such as 'old age', 'senior', 'elderly', 'retiree' and 'retirement' that are slowly giving way to a change in definition or other words such as 'rewiring' and 're-engineering'. Madeline Albright, the former US Secretary of State, is happy to call herself a perennial but not retiree or senior. Even words such as transitioning were not associated with retirement. Previously retirement just happened as we worked; the magical age of 65 arrived and we retired.

Two other alternatives to the meaning of the word 'retirement' are:

Maturation based on the Latin word 'maturare' meaning to ripen/ bring to maturity and is said to reflect both the financial and psychological aspects of this time of our life.

Jubalacion is a Spanish word meaning retirement. It is derived from the Latin word *jubilant* meaning 'to make a joyful noise'.

Social researcher, Hugh Mackay, in his book *Advance Australia....Where?* noted similar sentiments for Australian Baby Boomers to the word retirement. The image of elderly people living in nursing homes waiting for death seems to be deeply engrained in our minds.

Do you have a preference for how you would like to be referred to after finishing a lifetime of work?

Baby Boomers (or the 'countercultural generation') want to adopt a new generation identity in their post-retirement years because they are entering a new phase in their life. In the 1960s and 1970s, the Baby Boomers changed the world and have been doing so ever since. Now, with time and money at their disposal, what will they do in this next phase of their life?

At this stage, it might be worthwhile taking a brief look at the history of retirement and pensions...

The history of retirement, the pension and superannuation

From the beginning of mankind, the concept of retirement was unknown. People would start work at a young age and work until disease, accidents or wars killed them. If people were born disabled, or became incapacitated due to illness or accidents, then their family would provide for them. If capable, they became beggars relying on the generosity of other people. There was no need for an old age pension or retirement as, for most people, life expectancy was around 40 years. Those that did live longer were looked after by their family and were respected in their community.

Many people think that the pension, or something similar, is a relatively new concept. Surprisingly, a pension has been with us since Roman times. Since that time, many countries have provided a pension to the military and the police long before other members of the population were entitled to any such benefit. Even today, in many countries, members of our military and police forces are able to retire early, sometimes in their late 40s or early 50s, on a pension.

Prior to the Industrial Revolution in the eighteenth and nineteenth centuries, people lived in mainly farming communities where they could grow food for themselves and their dependents as well as trade any surplus for other items they needed.

From the industrial age onwards, there had been a major shift from the farms to towns and cities to obtain work. This created a reliance on other people for food and shelter. The factories were dirty and overcrowded and the work was hard and boring, resulting in many injuries and deaths. Later on, with the introduction of the production line, older workers were seen as detrimental to production; they were accused of slowing down the production line.

It was the German Chancellor, Otto Von Bismarck, who, in 1881, proposed that anyone over 65 years of age would be forced to retire and a pension paid to them. The pension was also paid to those disabled at work. It was proposed that the scheme would be mandatory and required the employee, the employer, and the government to contribute. The retirement age selected was 70 which aligned closely with the life expectancy at that time in Germany. It took eight years before the retirement scheme was created and there was strong opposition to it.

In other parts of the world, retirement ages and pensions progressed more slowly on a national level. In the United States, pensions were introduced primarily on an industry basis. The Social Security Act was passed in 1935 setting the official retirement age at 65. Around that time, the life expectancy for American men was 58 years.

There were some interesting thoughts being expressed in the late 1800s and early 1900s regarding age and retirement. William Osler, a Canadian physician giving the valedictory address to the John Hopkins Hospital in 1905, said that a man's best work was done before he was 40 years old and that he should retire by age 60. Workers in this age bracket 40–60 were tolerated because they were 'merely uncreative'. After 60 he said, the average worker was useless and should be put out to pasture. Thankfully, today's society has a different outlook to this.

In the colonies of Australia, care for the elderly and infirm was the responsibility of family, charitable or religious organisations or, in the worst case, government asylums for the mental and destitute. Around 1900, New South Wales and Victoria introduced state-based age pension schemes and Queensland followed in 1908. These schemes were replaced by the *Commonwealth Invalid and Old Age Pensions Act* on 10 June 1908 but it wasn't until December 1910 that the pension was paid.

The old age pension was payable to men from age 65. Following changes to the Act, from December 1910 it was payable to women from age 60, providing they were 'appropriately qualified people'. Average life expectancy for males around this time was 55 years and, for females, 59 years. Only about four per cent of the population was over the age of 65.

To receive the pension of £6 per annum, the person's income from other sources had to be less than £52 per annum for the pension not to be reduced. There was also an asset test where total assets, initially including the family home, could not exceed £310. (The family home was excluded from the asset test within about two years). There was a residency requirement, initially 25 years but reduced shortly afterwards to 20 years. The person also had to be of good character although what was 'good character' was not defined. However, a person who had deserted their spouse and children within five years was not eligible. Asians not born in Australia and Aboriginal and Torres Strait Islander people were also not eligible. The Commonwealth scheme followed closely the New South Wales scheme. A single pensioner received £0.10.00 (ten shillings) a week while a married couple received £0.15.00 per week.

In Australia, the pension remained relatively unchanged from 1910 until after World War II. However, since that time, almost every government has tinkered with the pension. It is worth looking briefly at some of these changes since World War II and how they have shaped our current scheme...

For a nation recovering after World War II, the Chifley Government made it easier for people to obtain the pension. During the Menzies era, property ownership exemptions were increased and then the Gorton Government introduced a tapered withdrawal rate. Older pensioners were exempted from the means test by the McMahon Government and Whitlam Government. The Fraser Government abolished the asset test entirely.

The biggest changes since 1910 occurred under the Hawke Government. Hawke and Treasurer Keating realised that the number of Australians receiving the pension had ballooned. They realised that there were too few workers supporting too many Australians receiving the pension and that this was unsustainable in the future. Initially, the Hawke Government introduced changes to the treatment of investment income, compensation payments were assessed, and assets were means tested.

But bigger and lasting changes were still to be introduced. In 1988, compulsory superannuation was introduced. At that stage, it was three per cent of gross income. Since that time, it has been gradually increased to the current 9.5 per cent with a target of 12 per cent.

The constant tinkering by various governments has resulted in a complicated but highly successful retirement income scheme.

Our parents and grandparents worked all their lives dreaming of things that they may do in their short retirement years; for example, that overseas holiday. Today, we can have many dreams spanning far more years.

For Boomers

Retirement is dead, long live retirement! Ok, I have played on 'The king is dead, long live the king' but, just as this was said as a king died and an heir was crowned king, so retirement as we have known it is dead – but a new retirement is alive. The new retirement is very different from the past. Retirement for many Baby Boomers will be longer, and more satisfying, than for many past retirees. It will be different, very different, for most people. Never before has there been so many people entering retirement and continuing in retirement for maybe 30 or 40 years.

It is also a time when retirees, pre-Baby Boomers, are still alive and living on a pension or their own savings and investments. So we have retirees who may have been through The Depression and World War II who have been very careful with their finances and we also have retirees, the Baby Boomers, who have been a very wealthy generation and been able to enjoy the good things in life.

The one constant since the original Australian pension was introduced in 1910, has been the philosophy that if you have the assets and income to support yourself in your old age then you will not be entitled to a government pension. The pension is the safety net providing a very basic level of income.

The Boomers have had a tradition of being non-conformists and this is continuing as they get older. They are dictating at what age they will retire; some may retire in their 50s whilst others may not retire until in their 70s, if at all.

However long the retirement, the common goal for most retirees is to live a long, happy and healthy retirement without money worries. For the Boomers, it is a new phase in their life with exciting times ahead.

To assist readers with this, the remainder of the book looks at many aspects that need to be considered both before retiring, and in retirement. Pre-retirees tend to focus much of their attention on their finances without considering what their lifestyle might be like. Yes, the financial aspect is important because nobody wants to be stressing over money in retirement. There are also many other aspects such as health and psychology that need to be considered in order to enjoy retirement.

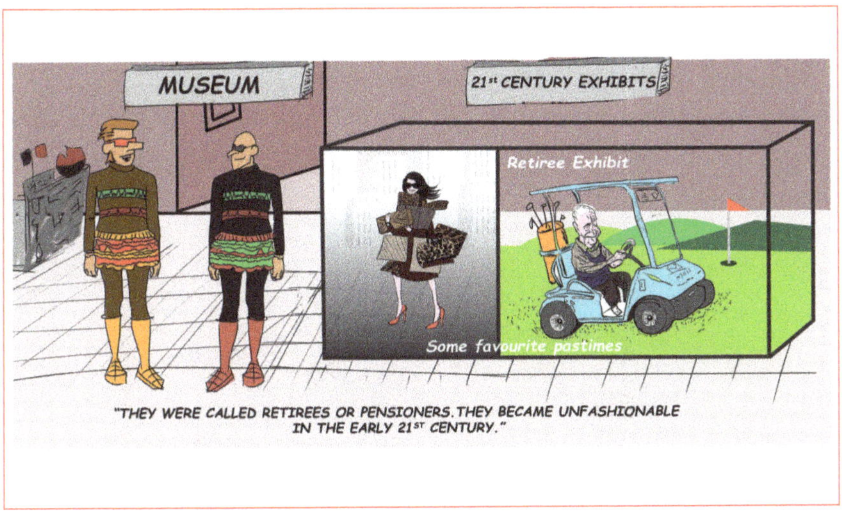

Post Boomers

Unfortunately, any crystal ball is likely to be very hazy on retirement for the Gen X and Gen Y. As the Baby Boomers retire and the workforce decreases, it is unlikely that a pension funded by the Commonwealth Government as we know it today will be available. Already we know that Australia, like a number of other overseas countries, has increased the retirement age for those born after 1 July 1952. The retirement age, or age at which you are eligible for a pension, increases by six months every two years until 1 July 2023 when the qualifying age for the pension in Australia will be 67 (as shown in the table).

Date of Birth	Age Pension Eligibility age
Before 1 July 1952	65 years
1 July 1952 – 31 December 1953	65 years and 6 months
1 January 1954 – 30 June 1955	66 years
1 July 1955 – 31 December 1956	66 years and 6 months
From 1 January 1957	67 years

There has also been a change to the preservation age for access to superannuation: for those born after 1 July 1964 to age 60. (The preservation age is the minimum age that a person must reach before they can access their superannuation). Superannuation funds can be accessed once the age of 65 is reached or the person is permanently retired and has reached the preservation age of 55 – 60, depending on the date of birth. The following table shows that the increase starts for those born between 1 July 1960 and 30 June 1961 and increases yearly until 1 July 1964. From there it remains at 60 for those born in subsequent years.

Date of birth	Preservation age
Before 1 July 1960	55
1 July 1960 – 30 June 1961	56
1 July 1961 – 30 June 1962	57
1 July 1962 – 30 June 1963	58
1 July 1963 – 30 June 1964	59
From 1 July 1964	60

People are retiring at all ages, not just at 65, and for all sorts of reasons. Some may take early retirement due to a downturn in the economy then after a few years go back to work. Others retire from one profession, retrain, and then start work again in possibly an unrelated field. There is also a growing trend for people to work from home in home-based businesses such as Amazon, Airbnb or start up their own consultancy business. There are also anti-discrimination laws now that prohibit discriminating against a person because of their age. Therefore a person can work as long as they wish. The economic conditions of the country, or in a particular state or territory, may also influence whether people continue to work or retire and possibly re-enter the workforce at a later stage.

Today, retirement could be as long as 20 or 30 years so retirees who are generally in good health can enjoy a greater variety of activities.

Whereas in the past retirement had been age-based, today it may depend on financial independence with people in their early 40s or 50s choosing to retire. In a later chapter we will look in depth at how people can, and are, reinventing themselves in retirement.

The first of this new wave of retirees, the Baby Boomers, turned 65 in 2011 so the majority of Baby Boomers are still to retire.

Why do you want to retire?

This is a relevant question to ask yourself. Is it because friends and colleagues have reached, or are about to reach, 60 or 65 and have retired? Maybe more importantly, do you want to retire? Even though you may be frustrated by work and long to retire, work has been a major part of your life. You have been conditioned from a young age that you will get an education and then go to work. Over the years, work has provided fulfilment and satisfaction, sometimes dissatisfaction, and a sense of belonging. This may, in part, explain why some people find it difficult to retire. Also, governments around the world such as Australia, Britain, Germany, Iceland, Norway and the United State of America, are all raising the pension age as they try to delay people retiring.

Many people start thinking about retirement from age 40-50. Many may come to understand how ill-prepared they are financially and this uncertainty can lead to anxiety and depression.

One way to help deal with the anxiety and depression is to identify what retirement might be like and then to practise this lifestyle. What may a typical month in retirement look like for you? Fill out the following four-week calendar with what you might do, whom you might visit, and any trips you might undertake. (This is not during a holiday but a typical month in your retirement). If you have a couple of weeks of leave available and no actual holidays planned, why not try putting two weeks of your typical month into practice. This may help to crystallise what your real needs are against your wants or wish list. You can then approach retirement with more certainty.

Typical Month						
	Monday	Tuesday	Wednesday	Thursday	Friday	Saturday	Sunday
Week 1							
Week 2							
Week 3							
Week 4							

There is no specific time at which people have to retire; a person could retire at 40 or 50 if they wish or maybe never retire. The big constraints are whether a person will be healthy, psychologically prepared and have sufficient funds to be able to live comfortably for the next 30 or 40 years.

The main reasons why people aged over 45 retire.		
	Men	Women
Reached eligible pension age	40	19
Sickness, injury or disability	19	14
Retrenchment, Dismissal or no work	9	6
Care for ill or disabled parent or partner	2	5

The Australian Bureau of Statistics reports that 1 in 4 Australians over 45 years of age, who intend to retire, expect to do so at age 70.

Between 2009 and 2013, the average age for Australian men retiring was 63.3 years and 59.6 years for women.

Sometimes retirement is forced upon us. The company that we have worked for is forced to downsize and we are faced with redundancy or retrenchment. Some even close their doors and it may be difficult to find suitable employment again. Sometimes ill-health of you, your partner or a family member may bring on retirement. Such forced and unplanned retirement can have long-term effects on the mental health and well-being of those retirees.

For others, they come to a realisation that now is the time that they should retire; maybe not immediately but within a relatively short timeframe. Deciding when to retire is best done jointly with a partner as it is likely to put pressure on the relationship, particularly if there are different expectations.

The following chapters will provide some clarity around this quandary...

How to retire

Since there is no age at which workers must retire, the lead-up to retirement has also changed dramatically. When there was compulsory retirement at age 60 for females and 65 for males, workers reached retirement age and basically stopped working overnight. This is often referred to as the cliff-edge retirement – over the edge into oblivion.

Today, there is choice and a lot to consider. For some, there is too much to consider. A cliff-edge retirement is always possible but many now select the date for their retirement. It is no longer into oblivion but potentially a very rich and rewarding life. Alternatively, with the agreement of your employer, you may gradually reduce your hours of work, maybe working a 9-day fortnight then four days per week then down to three days per week as a phased-in retirement.

Some people looking ahead to the future may consider a portfolio where they have a mix of part-time work and consultancy work or self-employment or voluntary work.

It is important when choosing one that you consider how these options may affect you financially. Will it affect your superannuation payout, your own contributions or your employer's contributions?

It is not uncommon, nowadays, for people to have a false start into retirement. They may have retired early and find that their friends are still working so nobody is available to join them for a long lunch or to play golf. After a period of time, they decide that they are not ready to retire. They then return to work either full-time or part-time until they feel that they are now ready to retire.

As a society, we have not yet developed appropriate norms for retirees. It is an opportunity for further self-development, new learnings, new challenges and new parts of the world to explore. As there are no norms, we should feel free to develop our own.

Preparation is the cornerstone to a happy retirement. We need to prepare emotionally, physically, psychologically as well as financially. We need a positive mental attitude, an ability to handle change and a determination to get on with the rest of our lives.

Chapter 2

Where are you currently?

Alice came to a place where there were many roads. She stopped and asked the owl for directions. The owl asked, 'Do you know where you want to go?' Alice said, 'No'. 'Well then', the owl said, 'it doesn't make any difference which path you take now!'

Lewis Carroll, *Alice in Wonderland*

In order to plan for a successful retirement, you need to understand where you currently are. What does retirement mean to you? What is the starting point for your journey of retirement?

It is very important that you are honest with the answers that you give in this assessment of where you are currently. The old saying of 'garbage in, garbage out' is true here. We will look at a number of assumptions as we progress, ie what inflation and interest rates might be, little change occurs to our superannuation or pension entitlements, etc. Unfortunately, these can only be guesstimates so your potential outcome will be improved if you can be as accurate as possible.

As you work your way through this book, you will find that it is far more than a book on finances. We have adopted a holistic approach to planning for retirement. In this chapter, we will also look at other important aspects in preparing for retirement. So let's begin by looking at some of these other areas of your life and then we can come back to our finances...

What will your life look like in retirement? What kind of life do you want to live? It is a tremendous opportunity to try new things, visit new places and live your dreams.

Health

We have placed health as our first topic to discuss because we believe that your health should take first priority in any discussion on retirement planning. Your health is a major determining factor in whether you can or cannot continue to work. This is important for everyone but particularly for males who generally have a poor attitude to health and visiting the doctor. When was the last time that you went to the doctor for a check-up? When was the last time that your doctor ordered a set of blood tests to check your cholesterol level?

How is your Body Mass Index (BMI) and your weight? As in most developed countries, many Australians are overweight or obese. Are you carrying fat around your stomach area? As we age, the type and amount of food that we need changes. Have you spoken to your doctor or dietician? If your weight is within acceptable limits it may be that you do not need a dietician, only a food nutritionist. Do you have a balanced intake of food – fruit and vegetables, fish and meat? How much water do you drink in a day and how much alcohol? Why not keep a track of what you eat and drink for a week or two – and don't forget the snacks. The results may surprise you. We are certainly not trying to take all the enjoyment of food out of your life but we do want you to understand what you are currently eating and how this may affect your life now and into the future.

When was the last time you visited your dentist for a check-up and a clean? Unfortunately, our Federal Government doesn't see dental health as being important enough to be part of Medicare. But poor dental health can lead to serious health issues.

Exercise is an area that is often misunderstood. As we age, it is important that we not only exercise sufficiently but that we exercise correctly. What exercise do you do? Over the years, many of us have become 'couch potatoes'. At work, many of us in professional or clerical positions spend a large amount of time sitting. We may walk to and from public transport or our car to get to and from work, maybe out for a coffee or to buy lunch, but when we get home we sit in front of the television. We no longer have to get out of our armchair to turn the television on/off or to change channels; we just point the remote control. Do you do any gardening? Do you walk and if so how many times a week and for how long? Is it a leisurely stroll with friends or do you actually get your heartbeat up as you walk briskly? Some of us may go to the gym but has anyone designed the gym program for your needs or have you just been shown how to use certain machines? Do you do any core strength or balance exercises? How flexible are you?

The food that our parents and grandparents ate was very basic; meat and three vegetables was a classic English meal and often with lard or dripping. Exercise was mainly walking and working around the house, not fancy machines at a gym. Unfortunately, their retirement years were generally relatively short. We now have a choice.

The food that you eat and the exercise that you undertake have serious implications for your health with potential issues such as diabetes, heart attacks and osteopenia to name a few. The sooner you start to look after your health, the better; it is often easier when you are younger to make the necessary changes.

How is your current exercise and eating plan? Have you been putting on a few extra kilograms? Do you need to change the amount you exercise or modify what and how much you eat? As we age, we need smaller portions and to eat more regularly.

Importantly, how healthy are you? If you are comparing yourself with work colleagues or friends, this could be very misleading. Ask your doctor for a complete checkup.

How would you rate your health?										
Fitness	1	2	3	4	5	6	7	8	9	10
Balance	1	2	3	4	5	6	7	8	9	10
Exercise	1	2	3	4	5	6	7	8	9	10
Weight	1	2	3	4	5	6	7	8	9	10
Diet	1	2	3	4	5	6	7	8	9	10
Memory	1	2	3	4	5	6	7	8	9	10
Mental exercise	1	2	3	4	5	6	7	8	9	10
Regular visits to the doctor	1	2	3	4	5	6	7	8	9	10
Regular visits to the dentist	1	2	3	4	5	6	7	8	9	10

Social

Often overlooked in the lead-up to retirement is how we socialise. We all have friends that we socialise with but how broad is your circle of friends? Who do you socialise with the most? These may seem unusual questions but, as you get older, it is important to increase your social circle. As your friends retire and get older, they may move to another suburb, town or even interstate. Some may die.

The broader your social network, the more enriched your lives will be and the longer you will have friends to socialise with. Your broad social network needs to include people of different ages and different interests.

It is important that you socialise with people other than your workmates. After retirement, it will only be a select few that will remain in contact and generally only if you have some other things in common. The days of going to the pub for a few drinks and talking about your boss or other workmates, or how the company and the country could be run better, will gradually lessen after retiring because you will have less in common. New people will have joined the company and you won't be current with what is happening with the boss or the business. However, these work/social relationships are important in transitioning from work to a much broader social base.

Who do you socialise with outside of work? Men, in particular, find it difficult to develop new friendships. You may not be sure where to start in finding new friends? Make a list of what you currently do outside of work; for example, leisure activities, and exercise and community groups. Are there people that you see regularly walking their dog or at the coffee shop that you may be able to start up a friendship with?

Now is the time to be developing these social networks. You may not have the time to build strong friendships now but start making acquaintances that may develop into friendships over time, particularly when you have the time in retirement.

How would you rate your social position currently?										
Current friends	1	2	3	4	5	6	7	8	9	10
Friends outside of work	1	2	3	4	5	6	7	8	9	10
New friends in the last 12 months	1	2	3	4	5	6	7	8	9	10
Ease of making friends	1	2	3	4	5	6	7	8	9	10
Friends independent of your partner	1	2	3	4	5	6	7	8	9	10
Friends of various age groups	1	2	3	4	5	6	7	8	9	10

Family relationships

How is your relationship with family members? This can be tested at times, for various reasons, sometimes resulting in irreparable damage. As you will read in the next chapter, family relationships are very important.

Our most important relationships should be with our spouse, children, grandchildren and, if still alive, our parents. Secondary are our relationships to our siblings and other extended family members. Ideally, having good relationships with all our family members would be wonderful but, in reality, this is unlikely. New people coming into the family through partnerships or marriage, other relationships dissolving through divorce or separation and new additions with grandchildren, all make for challenging family relationships.

How are relationships in your family? Do you do fun things regularly as a family? Do you regularly have family dinners?

It does become difficult as each family member has a busy life and, when married, develop their own family activities and relationships. Children and grandchildren grow up quickly so it is important to spend time with them. Equally important is spending time with your parents because it is only when they are gone that you realise how little you may know about them.

What can you do to develop your family relationships?

How would you rate your family relationships currently?										
Partner	1	2	3	4	5	6	7	8	9	10
Children	1	2	3	4	5	6	7	8	9	10
Grandchildren	1	2	3	4	5	6	7	8	9	10
Parents if applicable	1	2	3	4	5	6	7	8	9	10
Siblings	1	2	3	4	5	6	7	8	9	10

Accommodation

As you think about retirement, where you live is likely to be discussed. Prior to retirement it is important to consider your options in terms of where you will live in retirement. We have devoted a chapter to looking at various options including living overseas, as some people do.

Are you happy to continue living where you currently do? Have you thought about a tree-change or sea-change or moving to an over55s village? There are many things to consider.

Are there maintenance items that need to be undertaken now before retirement? Are there changes that need to be made to your house to enable easier access or changes to the garden to make it easier to look after? What about construction of an entertainment area or a pool?

Is there a sentimental attachment to the house that the children grew up in? The five-bedroom house was ideal for the family but is it suitable just for the two of you now? How many bedrooms will you need in a new house or can you utilise your current bedrooms to provide some income through Airbnb or student accommodation?

To relocate is a major consideration. Financially, there are the costs associated with selling and buying like agent's fees and commission, solicitor's cost and stamp duty so often there is little financial incentive to downsize particularly if you wish to remain in the same area.

What about your friends and neighbours in the area? Moving away may mean that you will lose contact with them and you will need to develop new friends in your new area.

There is a lot to be considered regarding your accommodation both now and into the future. Some incorrect decisions can prove costly in many different ways and we will discuss these further in chapter 8.

How would you rate your accommodation position currently?										
Happy in current accommodation	1	2	3	4	5	6	7	8	9	10
May consideration renovations	1	2	3	4	5	6	7	8	9	10
May consider moving	1	2	3	4	5	6	7	8	9	10
Close to transport	1	2	3	4	5	6	7	8	9	10
Close to shops, cinema	1	2	3	4	5	6	7	8	9	10
Good network of neighbours	1	2	3	4	5	6	7	8	9	10
Close to family	1	2	3	4	5	6	7	8	9	10
House is too large	1	2	3	4	5	6	7	8	9	10
Potential for students or Airbnb	1	2	3	4	5	6	7	8	9	10

Employment

It can be difficult at times to think about retirement as your head is in work mode most of the time and there is little time to imagine your new future or to plan for it.

However, things can change quite quickly. At work, there can be a number of changes which may affect how you view work and retirement. These changes could include;

1. Changes in leadership – either your immediate manager or in company leadership
2. Changes in policies and the direction of the organisation
3. A restructure, downsizing, or even closure of the business
4. As a result of some of these, or even completely independently, there may be increased work demand, loss of morale or a change in the work culture to a more impersonal or authoritarian style.
5. Technological changes may affect your job and your attitude to work.

Can you relate to any of these?

Even if you are not planning to retire for some years, now may be the time to start considering your options.

If you have thought of doing some part time work in retirement, now is the time to retrain and make sure your skills are current.

How would you rate your employment position currently?										
Happy with current employment	1	2	3	4	5	6	7	8	9	10
Like to change employment before retirement	1	2	3	4	5	6	7	8	9	10
Plan to retire before 60	1	2	3	4	5	6	7	8	9	10
Plan to retire between 60 – 65	1	2	3	4	5	6	7	8	9	10
Plan to retire before 70	1	2	3	4	5	6	7	8	9	10
No plan to retire	1	2	3	4	5	6	7	8	9	10
Plan to work part-time in retirement	1	2	3	4	5	6	7	8	9	10
My skills are good	1	2	3	4	5	6	7	8	9	10
Need to upgrade my skills	1	2	3	4	5	6	7	8	9	10
Unlikely to gain promotion	1	2	3	4	5	6	7	8	9	10
Job security is strong	1	2	3	4	5	6	7	8	9	10
Possible to reduce days worked to four days per week	1	2	3	4	5	6	7	8	9	10
I have a list of lifetime goals	1	2	3	4	5	6	7	8	9	10
I have no plans for new activities	1	2	3	4	5	6	7	8	9	10
I have few leisure activities.	1	2	3	4	5	6	7	8	9	10

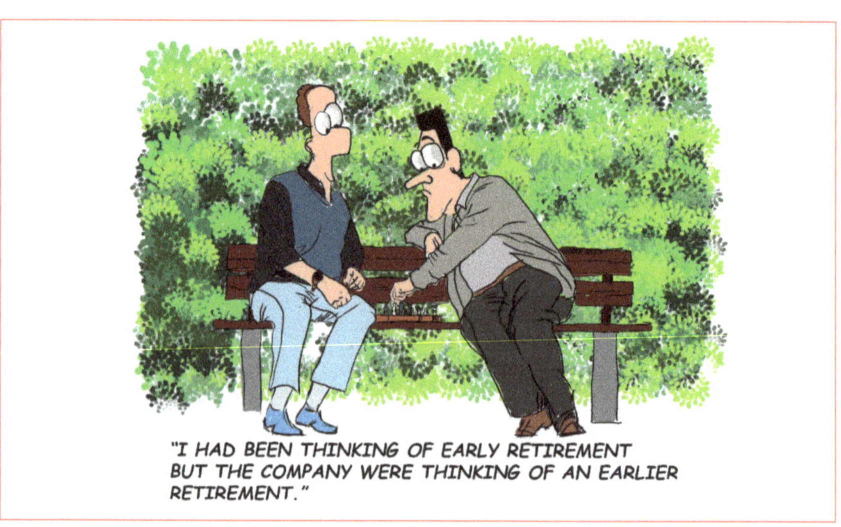

Leisure

You might have little time for leisure pursuits now, but in retirement, you will have time. What do you currently do now for leisure pursuits?

Do you like;

1. gardening,
2. to play a musical instrument,
3. to ride a bike,
4. to swim,
5. to read,
6. to dance, or
7. to travel?

How do you relax? Are there things that you would like to do if you had the time? Why not start now? You can start by making some enquiries, what groups may be in the area, who may teach languages or musical instruments, what community groups can you join and are there others in the area that you can share your passion with?

Do not wait until retirement to start thinking about any of these subjects. Take stock of where you are today, what you want to do in the future and start planning your ideal lifestyle. Dream like a child, without limitations.

Reflect on what has given you enjoyment and fulfilment in the past.

Start developing interests now (10 – 15 years before retirement) for what you want to do in retirement. Be realistic with where you are now and in what you would like to achieve.

How would you rate your leisure activities currently?										
I have active leisure activities	1	2	3	4	5	6	7	8	9	10
I plan to learn new leisure activities	1	2	3	4	5	6	7	8	9	10
I plan to travel around Australia	1	2	3	4	5	6	7	8	9	10
I plan to travel overseas	1	2	3	4	5	6	7	8	9	10
I plan to learn a new language	1	2	3	4	5	6	7	8	9	10
I plan to learn a musical instrument	1	2	3	4	5	6	7	8	9	10

Finances

Whatever type of lifestyle you want, your finances will be an important component of that lifestyle. Inadequate finances may mean that your dream lifestyle remains just a dream.

Most people tend to significantly under-estimate their retirement income needs.

As you prepare for retirement, it is important that you understand exactly your current financial position. Do you understand your risk tolerance? Are you prepared for higher risk in return for potentially greater returns from your investments? As you near retirement, your risk tolerance will change and you should be more conservative in your investing.

You probably know your income from your employment but what about any income from shares, rental property or bank interest?

Do you know the value of your property, share portfolio or superannuation and any loans against these? Do you have a plan to pay-down or pay-out any loans prior to retirement?

Are your income-producing assets structured to reduce your tax obligations? Arranging your affairs to minimise tax is prudent and perfectly legal. There is no moral or ethical reason why you should pay more tax than is required by law.

Have you maximised, or do you have a plan to maximise, your superannuation contributions?

Do you have adequate cash reserves or assets that can be readily liquidated or refinanced to redraw any available equity? Transitioning from a steady income in your working life to a passive income in retirement can be challenging.

Remember, every investment runs in cycles so be prepared by diversifying across different sectors.

While Australia's current inflation rate is 0.7 percent (September 2020 inflation rate) and Australia has had low inflation for the last decade, Australia's average inflation rate is approximately 3.2 percent.

Currently Australia has very low interest rates but in the 1980s and early 1990s, interest rates for over a decade ranged from 9.13 – 17 percent.

In the lead up to retirement, it is important to keep track of your expenses.

Transitioning from a regular employment income in working life to a passive income in retirement can be challenging. As you near your retirement date, have at least six months of living expenses readily available in cash.

An important part of funding your retirement is managing both your investments and your expenses to ensure that your funds last as long as they need to. Every choice you make now relating to your finances will have an effect on how much you have when you retire. Without some sacrifice and financial plan there can be no achievement of your retirement goals. It is the sacrifice you make today that will make all the difference when you retire.

It means not allowing your lifestyle to be dictated to by the income you earn. Do not spend it all – put some into savings.

The price of financial independence is eternal vigilance.

How would you rate your financial position currently?										
Prepare a budget	1	2	3	4	5	6	7	8	9	10
Review expenses regularly and make adjustments	1	2	3	4	5	6	7	8	9	10
Make additional superannuation contributions	1	2	3	4	5	6	7	8	9	10
Review insurances annually	1	2	3	4	5	6	7	8	9	10
Establish a regular savings plan	1	2	3	4	5	6	7	8	9	10
Invest for income	1	2	3	4	5	6	7	8	9	10
Invest for capital growth / wealth creation	1	2	3	4	5	6	7	8	9	10
Want security of capital	1	2	3	4	5	6	7	8	9	10
Want easy portfolio management	1	2	3	4	5	6	7	8	9	10
Have existing loans	1	2	3	4	5	6	7	8	9	10
Have a plan to pay-out or reduce loans	1	2	3	4	5	6	7	8	9	10
Seek professional advice	1	2	3	4	5	6	7	8	9	10
Review loans for best interest rates	1	2	3	4	5	6	7	8	9	10

Psychologically

Mentally, how are you feeling towards retirement? People have mixed feelings – some look forward to it and others are concerned. Those who have long defined themselves by their careers and position can find it difficult to feel relevant when they retire.

Have you reassessed who you are and found a new source of self-esteem? What is your purpose in life? A lack of purpose can lead to a loss of self-esteem, social isolation and time-consuming activities like drinking and gambling that do not contribute to your well-being.

Have you written down the things that you do well, listed your personality traits and those achievements that you are proud of?

Have you listed the things that you will miss at work and how you will replace them?

Many pre-retirees focus on the financial aspect but fail to think about, or prepare for, what their lifestyle in retirement might be like. The feelings of many people about retirement were directly associated with their financial position.

People who have a strong sense of identity embrace retirement more productively.

It is good to adopt an attitude of 'it's never too late'.

Give yourself time to adapt to pending changes.

Always make laughter part of your life. Years ago, the Reader's Digest published 'Laughter is the best medicine'. The more we laugh, the healthier we are so watch some funny movies or share a joke with a friend.

How would you rate your psychological position currently?										
I am looking forward to retirement	1	2	3	4	5	6	7	8	9	10
I am feeling anxious about retirement	1	2	3	4	5	6	7	8	9	10
I have established a new identity	1	2	3	4	5	6	7	8	9	10
I have good self-esteem	1	2	3	4	5	6	7	8	9	10
I am adapting to change	1	2	3	4	5	6	7	8	9	10
I laugh daily	1	2	3	4	5	6	7	8	9	10
I have structure in my day	1	2	3	4	5	6	7	8	9	10
I am ready for retirement	1	2	3	4	5	6	7	8	9	10
I have set a date for retiring	1	2	3	4	5	6	7	8	9	10

Key Learnings from this chapter

Chapter 3

Relationships

The best thing to hold onto in life is each other.
Audrey Hepburn

Humans, by nature, are social beings. Generally, we enjoy other people's company and this is particularly important as we age. Planning for retirement is the time to understand the importance of relationships and how relationships can and will change over time.

Each of us are different, some of us have long term and very close relationships with friends and family while others have a far less close relationship with most people.

In this chapter, we will look at our relationship with our spouse or partner, our children and grandchildren, parents and siblings and our friends.

Spouse or partner

Are you, your partner and your marriage ready for retirement?

This may seem a little strange to say particularly for people that may have been married for 30 – 40 years but you will need to readjust our lives in retirement. For the majority of your married life it has only been weekends and holidays that you may have been together 24/7. Now, you may have 20-30 years of togetherness 24/7. For some this may be ideal while, for others, it may be the beginning of the end.

Retirement can have some serious implications for your relationship with your spouse or partner regardless of how long you may have been together. We have previously mentioned that the divorce rate for those over 50 is increasing. That might well have a major impact on your retirement plans if not addressed early.

The lead-up to retirement can be a period of great change for both parties. Your body is changing, you may start to have some health issues, and you may now be empty-nesters. Now that you are starting to think seriously about retirement you must address the various concerns and feelings that may arise.

For those that have been married for a long period, there have been times when changes within the household have meant changes to the rules. For example, the birth of a child or when the last child leaves home. Retirement is also a new stage in the relationship so new rules need to be negotiated.

Regardless of how long couples have been together, many take their relationship for granted. It may no longer be seen as a priority with work and other commitments being seen as more important. Your conversations may decline and certainly what you talk about has changed. You need to think about what you and your partner generally talk about. It may revolve around how things went at work that day or, if there is a joint interest in some sporting event, what the result was and maybe some discussion on current events. It is no wonder that you get the comment from your partner – 'Are you listening to me?. Maybe you need to get back to the topics of conversation while you were courting to investigate true thoughts and feelings and to show a genuine interest in what your partner is saying. Over the years, you may have taken your partner for granted even to the extent of not noticing your partner's interests and desires changing over time.

Newly-retired individuals report the lowest marital satisfaction and highest marital conflict compared with those not retired, those retired for a long period of time and where both partners are retired.

There are many things that need to be discussed with your partner in the lead-up to retirement. Sometimes it may also be useful to discuss some issues with close friends as well as your partner, particularly if your friends have already retired.

Couples are genuinely worried about what they will talk about and do together in retirement and it is generally too late once retirement comes. You should start to develop both separate interests and shared interests and anything that goes along with those interests.

We will have a look at some areas that couples may need to consider…

One of the first areas that may need to be considered is the timing of your retirements. Do you both consider retiring on the same date, should the older person retire first, or should the wife retire first? Other factors to consider may be the health of each partner, the earning capacity of the partners or even the prospect of a redundancy package. Partners should play an important role in the retirement decision and each should feel they had some control over it.

There has been some evidence that it was better if the wife retired first but this may no longer be the case as wives are likely to be in positions that are just as stressful and earning similar salaries as their spouse. Females generally form new networks more easily than males and often then introduce their partner into the network; depending, of course, on whether the network is open to the spouse joining. It can also be very stressful for the wife, prior to her husband retiring, with concerns that he does not have much of a network and may spend a lot of time lazing around the house. The wife may then try to find things for the husband to do which can then be a source of tension.

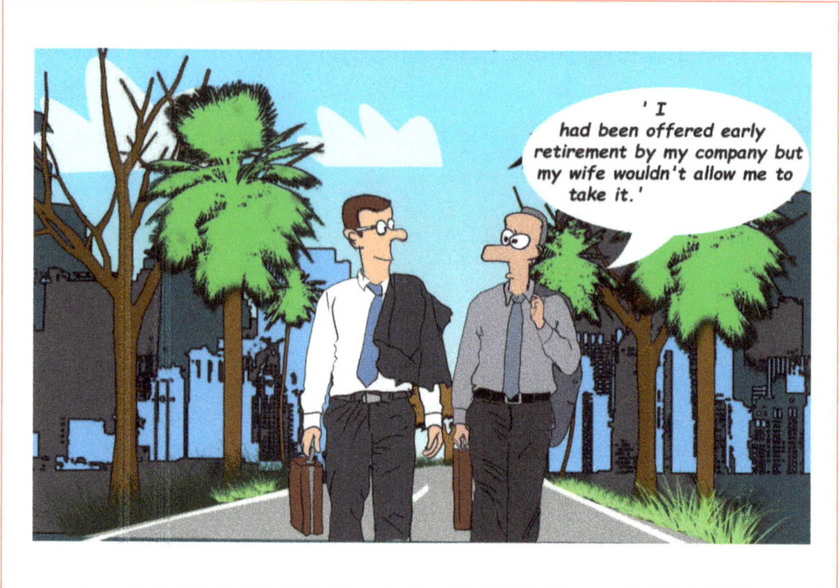

If one spouse does retire before the other, and takes on certain responsibilities around the house, then there needs to be discussion before the other partner retires as to how roles may change and even if they need to? The husband, for example, may have retired first and has undertaken the cooking, washing and house cleaning but when the wife retires she feels that, now that she has time, she can do a better job than her husband. Serious tension is created and needs to be resolved quickly – preferably before it starts.

A solid relationship, based on mutual respect and open conversation, will be more successful than one where trust, respect and communication are impoverished. It is very important to share decision-making through consultation and communication with your partner.

In our grandparents' day, the wife generally did not work, was often forced to retire when they married and therefore the wife's identity was tied very closely to her husband. The wife probably never retired as she continued her role of looking after the house for a long time after her husband retired from his employment.

Today, it is different with most partners working and developing an identity and status of their own.

It is therefore important that both parties consider each other and activities that they may undertake in retirement. If either party neglects the other's needs and interests, bitterness and anger is the likely outcome.

A couple may retire and leave their work environment but often, for the wife, the house is a secondary place of work where traditionally they have done the lion's share of the housework. This can still be the situation even if the husband has retired earlier and has undertaken most of the household duties while the wife was working.

Financial problems can be a major source of strain on a relationship at any time. It is particularly true in retirement when finances may be limited to one income or a fixed income from investments, or a pension. It is important that partners discuss any financial plans and decisions that are going to significantly affect their lifestyle.

The timing of retirement may be just one aspect of expectations of retirement. What other aspects may your partner have different views on? Who will take on specific roles such as cooking and cleaning, looking after the finances, planning holidays and allotting time for family and friends?

For those that have had managerial or supervisory positions, you need to learn that you no longer have staff and decisions need to be made with your partner on a consensus basis.

Have you spoken about your dreams and ambitions for the future? Have you shared the dreams of what your retirement might look like in the future? Have you discussed these with your partner and has there been any agreement? Over time, where there was once agreement, that may now have changed. This can be fairly common because, over the years, couples have developed a habit of living parallel lives, each busy with work and children.

Yes, both parties will need some time to pursue their own interests but what could you do together? It is important that each person has some independence but there will be things that you may want to do together. Have you developed a habit of sitting down together and planning the big picture including major holidays? In the past, time constraints may have resulted in this being delegated to one person but now is the time to devote time to work on things together. The ideal is to develop a balance between doing things that you both enjoy together and the time that you each have to pursue your own interests. It can be very disconcerting to find that your dreams and ambitions are so far apart or potentially in conflict with those of your partner.

Try some simple task together like going walking, going to the gym or maybe even some card or board games together. Another way is for each partner to prepare his/her own bucket list of what they want (not what they think their partner wants) to do. If you have been with your partner for any length of time, this may seem silly to say but don't make any assumptions about what your partner likes or dislikes. Once both partners have completed their list, compare the lists and develop a bucket list that you are both happy to work on for the next 10 years.

It is important to support your partner's interests. Things may have changed over time. The hobby or interest that only took a relatively small amount of time and resources could now occupy a large part of a day or week and require more resources, including money.

We have briefly mentioned it in the previous paragraphs without actually naming it but each partner needs their own territory. This may be the kitchen for the partner that is the chef, or the garden for the partner who has the green thumb. It may also be a room in the house that becomes that partner's sanctuary. That area is their space, it can be as clinically clean or as untidy as that person wants. It is their space so the other partner needs to respect that entry therein needs to be invited.

Sometimes there can be a sense of guilt by one partner towards the other regarding the amount of work being done. Providing each partner contributes their fair share to the household, either agreed or implied, there should never be any feeling of guilt. When the husband makes an appreciable contribution to domestic work around the house, marriages tend to be happier.

Finally, health can have a major impact on relationships so it is important to look after your health and that of your partner. Unfortunately, accidents and illnesses happen so consider how you, as a couple, may respond to such events.

Children

It is important to develop good relationships with your children. There are times, such as during teenage years, when the relationship can be tested but generally the relationship survives. As we age and our children become adults, we need to treat them as adults and confide in them when we are contemplating major decisions, particularly decisions that affect them. This could involve them in discussions about wills and powers of attorney, changing houses and retirement planning.

Your relationship with your children, and the relationship between the siblings, can also change when new partners come into the family. The family dynamics can change.

Blended families are now common in Australia so it is important to treat everyone equally.

Do you have any special family activities that all your children and their partners participate in such as a family dinner on the weekend or a designated day during the week? Do you have family holidays together? It is difficult as all members of the family may live busy lives but it is worth making the attempt to have this family time together – not just at Christmas.

Do you try to spend quality time with each of your children individually? Do you have shared interests and are there specific areas that one child can offer expertise or assistance with?

One thing that seems to bring parents and children closer together is the arrival of a grandchild…

Grandchildren

My wife and I are relatively new to grandchildren but we can now relate to comments such as 'more wonderful than they ever imagined, even better than having children'. Having your own children can be quite traumatic; sleepless nights, financial concerns with loss of income and, for your first child, a concern about the unknown. Becoming a grandparent also has some of these particularly the concern about the unknown. One of our friends who has a number of grandchildren gave us some advice: 'You know nothing'. While it seemed strange advice, it is true. Our attitude to childrearing changes with each generation as does the equipment required. We just bought a car seat for our grandchild and it is suitable for 0 – 4 years. In the first 12 months, the baby must be facing towards the rear of the vehicle. I cannot remember a requirement to have seats like this when our children were babies?

A few months after our grandson was born, his parents presented us with a wooden sign to hang in our house. The sign reads: "Grandma and Grandad's place where grandkids are spoilt and memories made". The night that they gave us the sign, we spent a long time talking about their memories of their grandparents. We have something to live up to. I have fond memories of both my grandparents. Both were very different in many ways but I learnt many things from them such as learning to tell the time from a clock face. The common theme was that both grandparents offered unconditional love in their own ways.

Times have changed and those approaching retirement have the prospect of spending maybe 20 or 30 years with their grandchildren compared to a far shorter time in previous generations. This is despite the fact that many families are now waiting longer to have children than in our time.

Another thing that has changed is an expectation that grandparents will become babysitters. Soaring childcare costs and, in some areas, difficulty in finding childcare places means that having grandparents who are willing to look after their grandchildren makes it affordable for both parents to work. It is difficult for parents, particularly the mother, to leave their children while they go to work. Being able to leave their children with a grandparent, who they know and trust will look after their child, makes leaving the child easier.

Looking after grandchildren can have some big benefits for the grandparents as well. It provides enjoyment, mental stimulation, motivation to keep fit and energetic and, for some, a new role to replace a loss of work identity. While I think most grandparents look forward to looking after their grandchildren, it is equally important not to commit too much time each week as you still have your own life to live. That may involve travel, simply meeting up regularly with friends, attending courses or volunteering. In the lead- up to retirement, when your time is limited, just being available at short notice can be beneficial but also do not be afraid to say that you are unavailable if you have prior commitments.

Today, your grandchildren can be interstate or overseas so you need to think how you may be able to keep in contact with them. Are they old enough to talk on the phone or should you *skype* them on a regular basis? If you are thinking of moving closer to your grandchildren once you retire, think seriously about the various scenarios and how they may affect you later in life. What may happen, for example, if you move closer to your grandchildren and in a few years' time, the parents and your grandchild have to move due to employment changes? You may not financially be able to follow them.

While there is one grandchild, it is easy to devote your time to that grandchild and build up a great relationship. But what about when a second, third or fourth comes along? It is important to spend quality time with each of your grandchildren even in the lead-up to retirement. How can you spend quality time with each of your grandchildren?

Another important thing for grandparents to remember is that there is another set of grandparents so they must be respectful of when they, too, can spend time with their grandchildren. Grandparents should also understand each other's position particularly when it comes to presents for the grandchildren. There should be no competition to outspend or buy multiple presents. Hopefully, the parents can provide some guidance to the grandparents in this regard.

Providing care for a grandchild is a 21st century version of the nucleus families of previous generations. We may or may not live under the same roof but the importance of the relationship between grandparent and grandchild is still very relevant.

Parents

In the lead up to retirement, many of us may still have parents that are still alive, living either in their own home or a retirement village. It is important to make time to visit regularly and, if practical, to take them out for a trip. It can be something as simple as taking them to the local coffee shop for a coffee and cake. Time spent can be rewarding.

It is also important that not only do you spend time with your parents but that they also get to see their grandchildren and great-grandchildren. This may need to take into account the parents' health and mental condition but as the *Old People's Home for 4 Year Olds* series on the ABC proved, there are a number of benefits for both the aged and the young to be gained from their interaction. A number of these older residents lamented the fact that they seldom saw their children or grandchildren.

If you are keen on family history, talking with your parents may be your last chance to gain valuable information about your grandparents and great grandparents. Too often we take things for granted. Even though I spent time with my parents, there were many questions that I have now that will remain unanswered like 'how and where did my parents meet?'. My father was born and raised in Scotland and the first time he came to Australia was on a Royal Navy cruiser. My mother was born and raised in Australia, had a trip or two to England to visit relatives so it was unlikely that they met in England. Do you have questions like this?

If you have siblings, let them know that you are taking mum or dad out for a coffee and give them the opportunity to do the same. While your motives may be pure, it is possible that your siblings may misconstrue spending time with your parents as a way of obtaining greater favour possibly leading to a larger part of any inheritance. It depends on the insecurity of your siblings.

The death of your parents and the subsequent division of inheritances can drive a large wedge between the siblings. Sometimes this is irrevocable so accept that and get on with your life. If your children still want to maintain contact with their nieces and nephews that is their decision and not to be interfered with.

Siblings

Maintaining contact with your siblings, even for close families, can be difficult because of busy lives and possibly living in different towns, states or countries.

While your parents are alive, you may get together for significant birthdays and at Christmas time but once your parents have died, contact with your siblings often becomes less frequent.

While maintaining contact with siblings would be ideal, it is not always possible and not the most important contact to maintain. The first priority for family relationships is your spouse, your children and your grandchildren.

Friends

As you enter midlife, your busy lifestyle generally takes its toll on your social network. Even when you are not working, weekends and some afternoons and evenings are taken up with children's sport so it is difficult to find time for social activities with friends. You may be lucky enough to meet every couple of months or maybe for drinks in the lead-up to Christmas. With a hectic work life and family life, it is little wonder that your network of friends decreases in midlife.

As you move towards retirement, it is also a time to start to reconnect with old friends. One reason for this is that we start to realise how important friendships are; often this realisation is brought about through the death of a friend or family member. Unfortunately, it is a sad stage of life that you are entering when people around your own age start dying. It is a sad reality but often makes a connection with people you have not seen for many years.

As you head towards retirement, it is up to you to make new friends and acquaintances and it will require some effort and imagination. This was not required with workmates as you were placed together by circumstance and a common interest of working for a company. There may have been some peer group pressure to conform and join social gatherings or there may have been an interest due to status or some mutual assistance in relation to your work.

As you near retirement, this may have less appeal as you are unlikely to want to climb the corporate ladder. If you are fortunate and have a good support network at work, it is likely that retirement will be harder to accept. This is particularly so with people in the military, police and emergency services where there is a strong camaraderie and regimented working environment.

In the lead-up to retirement and in retirement, your friendship network should grow and the quality of your friendships improves. Developing new friendships is one of the best ways to transition to retirement.

It is also likely that some friends may 'unfriend' you. This could be for a number of reasons but incompatibility covers a few of these reasons. The incompatibility may be because of a perceived economic gap between friends. For example, one couple has to strictly budget how they spend their pension while another couple travels overseas regularly. A second incompatibility can arise from an imbalance in friendships. For example, the wife may have a strong network of friends that remain during retirement but the husband's friends, which have been work-related, decline.

We have previously mentioned that it is up to you to develop new friendships but, for some, it is difficult. Here are some ways that you may find old friends as well as new friends...

Many schools will have school reunions. Some are held regularly, perhaps every ten years, while others are less regular. You may see your classmates in a different light – the champion sports person now walking with the aid of a walking stick, the dux of the school still needing to work because of poor investment decisions, the least likely to succeed now retired with a great family and living a life that many would envy. Do not be afraid of school reunions – people change, you have changed.

There may also be friends that you spent a lot of time with when both your families were young but they moved, or you moved, and over time you lost touch with them. Maybe, now is a time to reconnect with them.

If you like to travel, think about going on some escorted tours where you will meet new people with a common interest in travel. We have developed some long-term friendships with people from other countries that we met while on bus tours.

Are there regular events, classes or courses, where you meet with a variety of people? Can you look at developing a friendship with any of these people? Classes and courses provide a common interest and are a good way to meet a broad cross-section of people. Being part of a group that meets regularly makes it easier to form an opinion of a person over a period of time rather than making a quick judgemental call on a first meeting. Classes and courses, where a group has been together for some time, may be seen as cliquey and reluctant to allow a new person into their circle – but be persistent.

One reason people give for volunteering is to meet people so another area to form long-lasting friendships is with other volunteers and also those people who derive benefit from the services provided by the organisation.

It is crucial to develop friends of different ages because, as you have read, people die. Having some younger friends is healthy and should provide long-term friendships. Having a good peer group is also important particularly if some of your friends are slightly older and are already entering retirement or have been retired for a few years. They can be a good sounding-board to share your feelings, experiences and anxieties. As we get older, it becomes harder to meet people of different ages and different walks of life; so start early. You will benefit from having younger and older friends as they are likely to look at things from a different perspective. The tendency is to form friends with people around your own age so you have to put in the effort to find friends outside of your age bracket.

We have mentioned that you will lose friends due to death but it is also likely that friends will change due to illness, changing locations and sometimes their interests change. There are also friends that can become very negative about such things as their health, family and politics. It is acceptable to gradually unfriend these people if you don't want to associate with negative people.

I once read that old friends ground you in the past, new friends inspire and respond to your changing needs; they encourage you to try different things and forge new directions.

Is that not what we want as we prepare for retirement?

All relationships, no matter how long established, need work and consideration to flourish.

Did you know that how happy we are in our relationships has a powerful influence on our health? Retirees, and those planning for retirement that do not have a strong social network, have a much lower life satisfaction compared to those that do.

If we want to be healthy and enjoy our retirement years, does it not make sense to spend time developing good social networks before we enter retirement?

Relationships are important in our lives. Some of the benefits we gain from relationships include;

1. A sense of membership or belonging to a family group or a group of friends
2. Assistance at different times. For example, to provide transport if the car is being serviced or even physical assistance such as if you were moving house
3. An opportunity to help others in some way which in turn increases your self-worth
4. Friends and relatives acting as sounding boards for our opinions, concerns and feelings.

Key learnings from this chapter

Chapter 4

Financial aspects to consider

You can be young without money but you can't be old without it.

Tennessee Williams

A search of any search engine for the words 'retirement planning' will show finances in many of the result pages. We also see and hear conflicting media reports that we do not have enough money in retirement or that the average Australian does not have enough money to enjoy retirement. Most of us only have a vague notion of what enough money is.

In the media, we have all seen the headlines about how much money is required in retirement. Some organisations have gone so far as to divide the amount required into two levels: modest and comfortable retirement.

We suggest that there are two questions here but the question posed by many commentators and financial advisers is wrong. It may be easy to compartmentalise money required to meet the two categories above but it fails to take into account people's lifestyle or aspirations for the future. Also we often see figures quoted as a single or a couple. For a single person then whether they are male or female is also important. Females have a longer life expectancy than males but may also tend to have less in superannuation because of time out of the workforce with children and, in the earlier days, a lower salary.

Most companies associated with promoting retirement focus on the product but not the results that you seek in retirement. Their glossy brochures, charts and graphs promote their product but how many are interested in you and the lifestyle that you want?

We are all individuals and not everyone wants to go on overseas holidays or travel around Australia for twelve months. Even if we did, each of us would have different ideas of how we would like to do that: 5 star hotels, backpacker accommodation, destination, mode of travel? What do you want to do when you retire and who do you want to do things with?

The good and bad news for potential retirees is that Australians have one of the highest life expectancies in the world and this is forecast to increase over the next four decades according to the *2015 Intergenerational Report*. The bad news is that Australians are going to have to be able to fund this potentially longer retirement. In light of this potential longevity, early estimates that people could retire on 80 per cent of their final salary are now being revised to 100 per cent of their pre-retirement income.

The Australian Government is faced with a quandary. With a decreasing workforce (as the Boomers retire) but an increasing demand on available finances, does the government increase taxes or reduce services? This, in the long term, will be unsustainable leaving the government with few options. Cutting back pension payments or increasing taxes is likely to be unacceptable. Increasing the age at which we receive the pension or increasing the qualification requirements may be considered. We have already seen the Australian Government increasing the pension age to 67 by July 2023. A proposal by the current coalition government in 2019 to increase the age to 70 has been dropped, at least temporarily. (This proposal was not new as former Prime Minister John Howard tried it once suggesting we should work until 70 years of age). We must learn to support ourselves.

In 1992, the Keating government introduced the 'three pillars' approach to retirement income. The three pillars are: age pension subject to a means test, compulsory superannuation and voluntary savings through investments such as shares, property and additional voluntary contributions to superannuation above an employer's contributions. In September 2019, the Treasurer, Josh Frydenberg, announced a review of the three pillars approach.

Funding your retirement is not just about doing one thing just prior to retirement but doing a series of things throughout your working life. There are two main phases: the accumulation phase where you save and invest during your working life, and the drawdown phase in retirement where you live on your investments.

Despite all the media surrounding preparing for retirement, most people do not give much thought to organising their retirement, including their finances, until late in life. Little time, if any, is spent on preparing for other aspects of retirement such as health, leisure and relationships.

We believe that financial freedom in retirement is within the reach of most of us if we choose to go for it. Financial freedom has little to do with age. So what is financial freedom? We think that financial freedom is having enough money now to last us the rest of our life regardless of what activities we want to undertake and how long we may live. We are in charge of defining what kind of life we want. Once we have defined that life, it is a matter of putting together a solid plan to get there. But be aware that managing money is time consuming and stressful.

This is where the second question relating to 'how much is enough ?' needs to be answered. Some people are so focused on accumulating assets for their retirement that they lose valuable years of enjoying themselves in retirement.

One method of deciding how much we will need in retirement has been to pick an arbitrary number around 75–80 per cent of our current income as the amount required for our retirement income but there appears to be no factual basis for such a guess.

Another method is to record how much we need to support our current lifestyle and then add or subtract living expenses that may or may not be required in retirement. Our employment-related expenses such as business clothes, business journals, union fees, costs of getting to and from work may drop substantially but other costs may increase.

There are many promoters of schemes involving real estate, shares, forex trading and, more recently, cryptocurrencies aimed at providing a path to retirement but we will not look in any depth into these. (In the *It's My Time* series, there will be two books that look at residential and commercial real estate investments and another Blockchain, Cryptocurrencies & The Future which we recommend).

In the lead-up to retirement, there are a few things that we need to consider: where our income will come from, how we will spend that income, what will happen if we become unemployed, how much is needed to live financially free in retirement and how to make it last. Up until now, we have probably had a regular source of income from salary and wages. However, when we cease work where is the income to come from? Ideally, we should have multiple sources to our income stream. Now is the time to consider the possible sources of our income and how we may allocate that income.

But first, let us gain an understanding of our current status.

Sources of income now and into the future				
	Current Income		Estimated Income after Retirement	
Sources of Income	You	Spouse	You	Spouse
Salary /Wages				
Regular overtime				
Part-time work				
Bonuses				
Interest				
Dividends from shares				
Rental Income				
Savings plan				
Superannuation				
SMSF				
Pensions				
Reportable fringe benefits				
Other income				
Total				

Next you need to consider controlling our expenditure. You may or may not have prepared or used a budget in the past because you have had a regular income but with the prospect of retiring, and maybe not having a regular income, it is worth taking the time to look at our outgoings.

Often people think that budgets are restrictive, boring and even depressing. But this does not need to be the case. Budgets can be used positively. If money needs to be saved then a budget can identify areas for consideration. It will also highlight areas that need more attention for better money control. Budgets will also be useful for your accountant, finance broker or financial planner to understand your spending pattern and your financial position.

You can't predict what will happen with the economy in the next 12 months, let alone 20 or 30 years' time. Currently, you have low inflation at around 2 per cent, low interest rates but in the past, you have had deflation and high inflation as well as interest rates around 17 per cent in 1990-91. Hopefully, you will not see interest rates of 17 per cent again but you will likely see higher inflation rates and higher interest rates than at present. Whether you invest in the property or share market or both, over the years you can expect occasional corrections – the property and share markets will adversely impact on our financial objectives. You need to prepare a comprehensive strategy including time, our goals and objectives so that you can arrive at a comfortable living by our retirement date. Ideally, you should aim to achieve this a few years prior to our retirement date just in case you lose our job or there is a change in the economy, like a recession, which may affect our plans.

Delay retirement

The *Household, Income and Labour Dynamics in Australia Survey 2017* found that fewer people were retiring compared to over 15 years ago and that many people were returning to the workforce after a period of retirement. The survey found 28 per cent of men and 48 per cent of women in the 60-64 year age bracket were retired compared to 49 per cent of men and 68 per cent of women over 15 years earlier. Almost equal numbers of men and women in this age bracket were also returning to the workforce each year. In the 45-59 year age bracket, about 26.7 per cent of those having retired were now returning annually to the workforce.

Whether people can delay retirement or return to work after retirement is influenced by their health and, for a large number of Australians between 60-70 years of age, their health was reported as poor or fair. Predictions are that 1 in 4 men and 1 in 5 women in their 60s will have poor or fair health according to a 2015 AMP report, *Going the distance: Working longer, living healthier.*

Some people delay retirement so that they accumulate more wealth without actually having any idea of what amount is required. They are offsetting the accumulation of wealth against potentially good health and energy that they may be able to use in travel or in spending quality time with family and friends. But for others, building in some longevity to their career gives some greater flexibility with more time to plan their retirement.

It is acknowledged that not everyone wishes to retire and this appears to be a world-wide trend. Their work provides their identity, their sense of worth, their social network as well as regular income. For others, being able to work represents a determination to stay young. Too often a desire to continue to work is looked upon negatively. These people are often seen as having to work because they have not planned correctly for their retirement. Do we think that this is the reason why people like Warren Buffett, Rupert Murdoch or the Queen of England continue to work? Are they some of the people whose job satisfaction grows with age? It also appears that stress levels are lower as people age.

Age pension

We do not plan to go into a lot of detail here on the age pension or any other pensions as it changes frequently and there are a number of variations. We will, however, cover the main areas relating to eligibility such as age, income test and asset test so that you can assess whether an age pension is likely to be part of your retirement plan. Over a number of years, I have seen retirees spend or gift a significant part of their retirement savings in order to be able to qualify for the pension. They do this so that they can qualify for the Health Card and associated benefits. One would have to wonder how much the Australian Government would save if the Health Card and benefits were given to all who reached pension age rather than having retirees using their superannuation and other savings on overseas trips, house renovations etc., to qualify under the asset and income tests.

There is a residency requirement to be eligible for the Australian Age Pension which requires an applicant to have been an Australian resident for at least 10 years – not necessarily continuous except for the last five years in which there must be no breaks in residency. There are some exceptions such as refugees or former refugees and people who have been receiving a partner's allowance, widow's allowance or widow B pension. They can transfer across to the age pension without meeting the residence rule. If a person is a female whose partner has died while both were Australian citizens then the eligibility requirement is two years before making a claim. If Australia has a social security agreement with a country that the retiree had lived or worked in, then they may also be able to claim.

Eligibility for the age pension is currently 65 years and 6 months and is set to increase to 67 by July 2023. A proposal to increase it to 70 by 2035 by the Turnbull Government has been reversed, for now. The same age limits apply to both men and women.

Age pension age requirements	
Born between	Eligible age
1 July 1952 to 31 December 1953	65 years 6 months
1 January 1954 to 30 June 1955	66 years
1 July 1955 to 31 December 1956	66 years 6 months
From 1 January 1957 onwards	67 years

The Australian Government applies an income test for people receiving the age pension, wife pension, widow B pension, bereavement allowance, carer payment and disability support pension. If a person is classified as permanently blind then the income test does not apply for the age pension and disability support pension unless they are receiving rent assistance.

For couples, the combined income is the same whether they are living together or apart due to ill-health. There are some transitional rates and variances if you receive a work bonus which will not be covered here.

Age pension income test 1 July 2020 – 30 June 2021	
Income per fortnight	Pension reduction
Single person	
Up to $178.00	No reduction
Over $178.00	$0.50 for each dollar over $178.00
Couple – combined income	
Up to $316.00	No reduction
Over $316.00	$0.50 for each dollar over $316.00

For retirees considering an age pension, they need to understand how the deeming system works. As retirees could have investments spread across multiple individual investments like different term deposits and different individual shareholdings, the government applies a notional interest rate known as the deeming rate to those investments regardless of the actual earning rates.

In 2019, with the low interest rates, pensioners have been calling on the government to review the deeming rates as they do not reflect the current earnings of pensioners.

The Australian Government also applies an asset test based on assets – property and items owned by the retiree or their partner fully or partially – or if the retiree has an interest in both Australia and overseas. The value of the asset is the market value after allowing for any debt secured by that asset. If an investment property was owned and worth $1,000,000 but had a mortgage of $800,000 then the assessed market value for the asset test would be $200,000.

A person's principal place of residence, their home, is exempt from the asset test. If living on a farm, the family home and surrounding land up to 2 hectares on the same title is exempt from the asset test. A person who sells their home with the intent of buying another will have twelve months in which to do so. Any interest earned on this money will be included in the income test. Some other exemptions include:

- aids for people with a disability
- granny flat rights where the person pays more than the extra allowable amount
- any property or money left as part of an estate and which can't be received for up to twelve months
- accommodation bonds paid on entry to a residential aged care facility
- cemetery plot and a pre-paid funeral or up to two funeral bonds subject to an allowable limit.

There are some rules covering granny flat and retirement village contributions which are too complex to cover here. There are also annual limits on assets that can be given away before the asset test will be affected.

Assets that are included in the asset test include:

- the market value of investment property
- financial investments
- superannuation
- business assets, if the retiree is a partner or sole trader
- motor vehicles
- boats and caravans
- household contents
- personal items such as jewellery, cameras and computers
- the surrender value of whole-of-life insurance policies

- hobby or investment collections such as artwork or wine
- cryptocurrencies.

If the retiree is a trustee of a trust such as a family trust or a director of a private company, some of the assets and income will be assessed.

Assets test limits are updated in January, March, July and September each year.

Age pension asset test 1 July 2020 – 30 June 2021				
	Full pension		No pension	
Marital status	Home-owner	Non-home Owner	Home owner	Non-home Owner
Single	$268,000	$482,500	$585,700	$ 800,250
Couple	$401,500	$616,000	$880,500	$1,095,000
Couple separated by illness	$401,500	$616,000	$1,037,000	$1,251,500

Age Pension Maximum Payment Rates per Fortnight 20 March 2021 – 19 September 2021			
	Single	Couple combined	Couple living apart due to illness
Basic rate	$868.30	$1,309.00	$868.30
Pension supplement	$ 70.30	$ 106.00	$ 70.30
Energy supplement	$ 14.10	$ 21.20	$ 14.10
Total	$952.70	$1,436.20	$952.70

Therefore the annual pension for a single is $24,770 and $37,341 for couples as at 20 March 2021. The age pension is taxable income and is added to any other income earned during the financial year. After allowing for various offsets and other credits that may be available, a single retiree is likely to pay no tax on an income up to around $33,000 and around $29,000 each for a couple.

There are transitional rates for people getting part-pensions on 19 September 2009 until they catch up with the current normal rates.

Over the years while an accountant and financial planner, I have seen many people go to extreme lengths in order to obtain the age pension or, in particular, the health card benefits. Some of the ways that they have boosted their pension or obtained the pension included;

1. Spending money on improvements on their house
2. Gifting to charities or family members up to $10,000 per year or $30,000 over a five year period
3. Overseas holidays such as round the world cruise
4. Prepaying funerals
5. Account based pensions and annuities that were not included in 'deemed income' calculations
6. Regularly reviewing the value of your assets; like your car and household contents. (Centrelink accepts the 'written down' value not the insured value of assets).

The Australian Government, like most governments in the world, is faced with unsustainable and increasing demands on the available finances. Governments have known for years of the tsunami of Baby Boomers due to retire. This means that there will be less revenue with a likely increase in pensions. In the years ahead, there is likely to be reviews of government pensions and benefits with potential cutbacks or increasing age requirements.

You may decide now that it is better to develop a plan to support yourselves so that you are in control of your financial independence and you therefore do not have to worry about the government pension.

We will now look at some areas that may be considered in order to maximise financial independence when transitioning to retirement.

Other Government Allowances
If a person is required to care for a person over 16 years who is disabled, is frail or elderley or has a severe medical condition

(your partner or parents), they could claim a carer allowance. This allowance is not subject to an income or asset test and is tax free.

There is also a carer payment and carer supplement which may be considered.

Maximise your salary

In the lead-up to retirement, it is important to maximise your salary by either a pay increase and/or by reducing taxes, and to put this towards savings.

One effective way to reduce taxation, if you are of preservation age, is to look at a transition to retirement (TTR) strategy. There are two benefits of this scheme: firstly it allows you to supplement your income while working less hours and, secondly, it saves tax.

To be eligible for the scheme, you must have reached your preservation age and be 55-60 to start the transition to retirement pension. Your employer will continue to make the superannuation guarantee contributions into the accumulation account of the superannuation fund and you need to set up an account-based pension account within the superannuation fund. The only limit on how much you can transfer to the pension account is that the accumulation funds need to remain open to receive the employer's contributions. Up to age 65, you can then withdraw between 4-10 per cent of the account balance each financial year as a pension income but not as a lump sum.

Once you have reached 60, your pension should be tax-free and, between 55-59, your pension payments are taxed at your marginal tax rate less a 15 per cent offset.

The Transition to Retirement scheme is good for those aged 60 or older and are in the middle to upper-middle income bracket.

Part-time work

While working, we may think that we do not have the time for part-time work or maybe do not have the need for part-time work.

In the lead-up to retirement, part-time work can provide some extra income to put into superannuation or to pay existing debts

Part-time work can be beneficial in retirement by providing additional income. It is also important for providing social contacts. It will be useful to look and try various options even though these options may not be related to your current occupation. One person found that stacking shelves provided some physical exercise and pocket money – quite different from the managerial position he previously held. Many employers have found that older workers have a better work ethic – they work hard, are punctual and have few sick days.

However, do not plan your retirement income on the basis of being able to obtain part-time work in retirement. If you think that you may work part-time in retirement, in order to improve your prospects of obtaining work it will be good to maintain or improve any skills that you may have – particularly computer skills.

Investment vehicles

This section on investment vehicles is just a snapshot of some of the advantages and disadvantages and is far from complete. It is recommended that you seek professional advice from your accountant or solicitor before making any choice of what is the most suitable business structure for you now and into the future.

Sole trader

This is the most common and simplest method of investing. The assets are owned by the individual, the debt is owned by the individual. Any income or profit is included in the individual's personal income tax returns and taxed at their marginal tax rate. If a large capital gain is made on the sale of the asset (after allowing for the 50 per cent CGT discount after 12 months), then the individual may incur a large tax bill. There is no asset protection if the individual was to be sued or become bankrupt. There is also no flexibility with the distribution of income nor with who pays tax on that income.

Partnership

This is where two or more people share ownership; commonly between spouses where they jointly own a house, an investment property or a business. The responsibility for running the partnership is shared and there is greater potential to share time, money and skills than as a sole trader. There may be taxation benefits and taxation is relatively simple. Tax is paid at each partner's individual tax rate although a partnership return is prepared. Any losses in the partnership are transferred to the individual's tax returns.

Like a sole trader, liability is unlimited with the additional complexity that each partner is jointly liable for the actions of the others in the partnership. The 50 per cent CGT discount is applicable to any asset sold after being held for 12 months.

Companies

A proprietary company requires a minimum of one director and one shareholder. The shareholders are the owners of the company but the liabilities of a company's shareholders are limited. The company pays tax on any profits at the company tax rate which may be lower than the shareholder's marginal personal tax rates. If the company pays a dividend to the shareholders, the shareholders may also receive a tax credit through the dividend imputation system for the tax paid by the company.

A disadvantage of a company structure is the initial establishment costs as well as ongoing costs such as annual fees and accounting costs. Also, any losses can only be offset against future income and a company is not able to obtain the 50 per cent CGT discount on the sale of investments after 12 months.

Trusts

A trust is an entity which separates legal control from beneficial ownership. Trustees control the day-to-day operation of the trust and any income or capital flows through to the beneficiaries. Trusts are promoted as an asset protection vehicle. Most trusts in

Australia last for 80 years with South Australian trusts being the exception to the rule.

The main roles and responsibilities in a trust are as follows:

A settlor is an independent person who initiates the formation of the trust and gifts the initial settlement sum. After the establishment of the trust and gifting of the funds, the settlor is no longer involved in the trust. If the settlor is, for example, a solicitor or accountant, they cannot invoice for the initial settlement amount – it must be a gift.

An appointer is given the power under the Deed of Settlement to appoint, remove and replace the trustees. In a family trust, a joint appointor is generally recommended as well as a clear succession if the appointor dies or becomes incapacitated.

A trustee can be a person or a company specifically incorporated for the purpose of acting as trustee. Trustees can be held liable for any actions undertaken in their capacity of trustee and, if a 'natural person', should always make it clear that they are acting in the capacity of trustee. The trustee is the legal owner of all property in the trust fund but these assets are held on behalf of the beneficiaries specified in the trust deed.

Beneficiaries are defined in the trust deed and can be up to three generations, for example, grandparents, parents, children and the extended family of these generations. For a discretionary trust, the beneficiaries have no entitlement to any income nor capital. Any beneficiary can be excluded from the annual distribution. The trustee has a responsibility to the beneficiaries to exercise discretion bona fide and in good faith.

There are basically three main types of trusts:

A *discretionary trust* is where the beneficiaries of the trust do not have any fixed or specified entitlement to the capital assets or income of the trust. The trustees can distribute any income or capital gains to any beneficiaries, often in the most tax-effective manner. Discretionary trusts generally do not pay tax as any income is distributed to the beneficiaries who then pay tax at their marginal tax rates. Beneficiaries, excluding companies, who receive any capital gains can claim the 50 per cent CGT discount if the asset has been held for more than 12 months.

A company can be a beneficiary of the trust and any distribution to the company would be capped at the company tax rate.

Unit trusts are often used where unrelated parties run a business or hold an asset such as property for development. A major difference from a discretionary trust is that unit trusts predetermine the unit holder's entitlements which may be for capital, income or both. A family trust can be a unit holder in a unit trust.

Hybrid trusts(less common) have taken the best features of both the discretionary and unit trusts to create a flexible tax planning solution. They are often used to gear into property but can be difficult to finance and costly to administer.

Superannuation

Since 1992, Australian employers have been required to make contributions to the employee fund through the Superannuation Guarantee. Originally 3 per cent, the current rate is 9.5 per cent with an aim of increasing that rate to 12.5 per cent by 2025.

In addition to this guaranteed amount, employees can also make voluntary contributions to the fund. Unless an industrial award specifies a fund or choice of funds, the employee can choose which superannuation fund they would like their contributions paid into. When choosing a fund, it is important to check the fees and costs of the different funds as these can vary widely. These fees ultimately affect the fund balance available at retirement. As well as the fees and charges, it is also important to look at what types of insurances are available; for example, life and disability insurances and their cost. You also need to compare what investment options are available, how the funds have performed over the last five years and whether you can swap or split your balances between the various investment options. There are a number of websites available to compare superannuation fund performances, fees and charges.

There are no maximum limits placed on lump sum or pension withdrawals but the government imposes minimum pension rates that you must withdraw each year from Account based pensions. The trustee converts some or all of the funds in the Accumulation fund into an account based pension which then pays a regular income. These minimum rates are set out in the following chart.

Note that 50 per cent of the minimum drawdown rates apply to the 2019/20 and 2020/21 financial years. The rates shown will apply from 2021/22 financial year.

Minimum pension rates to be drawn from superannuation		
Age range	Minimum pension as a percentage of account balance	$500,000 balance in account based pension minimal withdrawal
55–64	4	$20,000
65–74	5	$25,000
75–79	6	$30,000
80–84	7	$35,000
85–89	9	$45,000
90–94	11	$55,000
95 and over	14	$60,000

Income and capital growth within an account based pension is tax free and no tax is payable on any withdrawals by a person over 60. On the death of the member, the balance of their fund is tax free to their nominated dependent.

There are a few types of superannuation funds categorised as retail, industry, public sector, corporate superannuation and My Super (introduced by the Gillard Government in 2010).

My Super is an inexpensive, no-frills superannuation that acts as a default fund if employees do not choose a fund. There are restrictions on unnecessary or excessive fees, a ban on entry fees and commissions, and limited exit fees. There is a single diversified investment strategy.

Industry funds are membership-based mutual funds originally established for workers in specific industries. Many have now broadened their membership by allowing extended family members to become members. There are not-for-profit superannuation funds some of the best-known examples of which are SunSuper, UniSuper, MTAA Super, REST Industry Super, Hostplus, Cbus Super and Legal Super.

In contrast, retail superannuation funds are run by banks and insurance companies to generate profits for the company and ultimately a dividend to the shareholder. Many of these superannuation funds came in for criticism in the *2019 Royal Commission into Banking*. Examples of retail superannuation funds include AMP, BT, ING, MLC, Colonial First State and Suncorp.

Public sector funds were created for employees of federal and state government departments but some are now open to family members. Initially they were defined benefit funds and some older members may still have eligibility for the defined benefits. New employees are in the accumulation fund. Like industry funds, profits are returned to the fund for the members' benefit. An example is QSuper, for the Queensland Government.

Larger corporations operate their own superannuation fund under a board of trustees comprising members appointed by both the employer and employees. Some small to medium sized corporations have partnered with a large retail or industry fund to provide a corporate fund for their employees.

Superannuation is one of the most tax-effective ways to generate income in retirement but it is also very effective in wealth creation.

If you are to receive an inheritance or sell an asset, one option to consider is to contribute these funds into your superannuation. The current non-concessional contribution limit is $100,000 each financial year or using the bring forward rule, contribute $300,000 over three years.

If a person is over 65 and wishes to downsize their home, they can contribute $300,000 into their superannuation subject to the following;

1. Owned their house for at least ten years
2. Not be subject to CGT on the sale
3. Transfer the funds into the superannuation fund within 90 days.

For people aged 65-74, they can make superannuation contributions if they are gainfully employed for 40 hours within 30 consecutive days during a financial year that the contribution is made.

For those over 75, no superannuation contributions can be made unless it is a mandated employer contribution.

Those with larger fund balances may wish to consider a Self-Managed Superannuation Fund (SMSF).

Self-Managed Superannuation Fund

This is a private fund for (currently) up to four members. All members must be trustees of the fund and are responsible for all decisions and compliance with the relevant laws and regulations. Regulation of a SMSF is now the responsibility of the Australian Taxation Office (ATO).

A SMSF is a trust established for the sole purpose of providing for members' retirement. As at March 2019, there were some 598,429 SMSFs with more than 1.13 million members (source ATO).

Prior to establishing a SMSF, consideration needs to be given to the set-up costs and ongoing expenses which can be high, particularly for funds with small balances. Some of the ongoing expenses include accounting, tax, legal and financial advice plus an annual audit by an approved SMSF auditor.

Each SMSF is required to have an investment strategy that takes into account the members age and risk tolerance and can provide for members' retirement needs. One of the attractions of an SMSF is that members can choose from a broad range of investments for allocating their funds. Examples are:

* term deposits
* shares – both direct and managed funds
* property - both residential and commercial
* collectibles such as artwork, antiques, wine, vintage cars jewellery, coin and stamps
* cryptocurrencies (more recent).

Each has risks and specific rules regarding how they can be held. What you invest in, and the percentage of that investment compared to the total assets in your fund, must be within the parameters set in your investment strategy. In August 2019, the ATO advised that it intended to write to some 17,700 SMSF holders who had been identified as having more than ninety per cent of the funds in a single asset such as property.

In June 2018, findings into a review of the SMSF sector were released by ASIC. Two of the major findings were that 38 per cent found that running their SMSF was more time-consuming than expected and 32 per cent reported the set-up and running costs were more than they expected.

In the lead up to retirement, a pre-retiree should seek professional advice regarding a superannuation re-contribution strategy. The strategy involves withdrawing part of your superannuation and then re-contributing it back into the fund as a tax free non-concessional contribution. One little known benefit of this strategy is that it reduces tax payable in the event of the retiree's death and the superannuation funds passing to non-dependents such as adult children. Any taxable portion of the fund would be taxed at 16.5 per cent.

Investment options

Any investment planning should take into account the improving longevity of retirees meaning that growth as well as income-producing assets needs to be considered. The years before retirement are important years and the key to building a significant retirement benefit is to start accumulating money and assets early. Time then allows compound interest to work most effectively. As your income increases make sure that your level of savings also grows. Too often, our income increases but so too does our expenditure and level of debt. This is not the time for your debt to be increasing.

Savings plan

Many people think that they can rely on their superannuation. This is important but you also need to develop a savings plan. You may have had a regular income but this will change once you retire. This loss of income can be daunting and stressful for many people so now is the time to start preparing. Having a cash buffer will relieve some anxiety, knowing that there is an amount to fall back on. How large that cash buffer needs to be is an individual question. Are there any fixed expenses such as mortgage, rates, insurance, car repayments and health insurance? If so, consider a buffer which includes these amounts for a 6 or 12 month period.

You may expect to receive a lump sum when you leave work but we have suggested a regular savings plan as the means to build up your cash buffer. This will serve a twofold purpose; it will build up your cash buffer but also reduce your immediate spending power thus helping you to live a simpler lifestyle.

Bonds

In purchasing bonds, you are lending your money to the Australian, state/territory governments or large corporations at an agreed interest rate for an agreed period of time. The interest is paid at regular intervals, normally half yearly or quarterly, and your loan amount is repaid in full at the end of the period. Some terminology associated with bonds is:

* face value is the amount you will get back on maturity
* coupon rate is the interest paid each year
* a green bond refers to the 'green' types of projects that the funds will be used for such as renewable energies, environmental benefits or social responsibility.

The interest rate can be fixed or floating (variable). Fixed interest rates are set when the bonds are issued and expressed as a percentage of the face value of the bond.

Bonds have been seen as a defensive investment as some perform well when the market is struggling. For example, a 10-year bond may have been purchased with an interest rate of 5 per cent per year. If the interest rate then dropped to 2.5 per cent, the income from your bond would be twice as valuable as others and the price of the bond would increase. Unfortunately, the reverse can also happen.

Bonds are traded on a secondary market such as the Australian Stock Exchange and are known as listed or exchange-traded bonds; most have a credit rating.

Debentures

Unlike bonds, debentures, secured and unsecured notes are unlisted investments and so cannot be traded on a secondary market like the Australian Stock Exchange. Companies issue debentures, secured and unsecured notes to raise funds from investors in return for regular interest payments. Details of the debentures such as loan terms, interest rates, reasons for borrowings and any security are set out in a prospectus. Debentures have tangible property as security while secured notes have first-ranking security over other property; unsecured notes have no security. The period of the loan varies from 1, 3, 6 or 12 months up to 5 years and unless the debentures are referred to 'at call', the loan period is fixed. Often the loan period can be extended by rollover and can happen automatically if you do not advise the company that you wish to have your debenture repaid.

Exchange Traded Funds (ETFs)

These are another type of managed fund that can be bought and sold on a securities exchange market. ETFs cover a broad range of assets including shares, fixed income products, foreign currencies, precious metals and commodities. If the ETF buys the underlying investment such as shares, it is known as a standard or physical ETF. The main risk is the performance of the underlying asset. In contrast, synthetic ETFs have a material exposure to derivatives as well as the underlying assets that the ETF is tracking. The derivatives add additional risks such as credit risk.

A passive ETF tracks an asset or market index without trying to outperform the market. On the other hand, the fund manager of an active ETF tries to outperform the market or index.

Some of the main risks associated with ETFs are that market liquidity can make ETFs harder to sell in certain circumstances and they are more complex and volatile than ordinary company shares. If the ETF has overseas assets, then there is a currency risk associated with the Australian dollar. Some ETFs reduce this risk by currency hedging. ETFs located in other countries may also be subject to foreign taxes.

Fixed interest or term deposits

This is typically when you place money in the bank for a fixed term and interest rate.

Annuities

Sometimes referred to as a guaranteed annuity, it is another form of income stream. There are two main categories; lifetime annuities which pays an annuity for the life of the recipient and specified period annuities which pays an annuity to a specified date.

In addition to the two annuities mentioned, there are a number of options that can be added to the type of annuity chosen. One option is a reversion where the partner is entitled to a nominated percentage of the payment when one partner dies. The second option is escalation where the annuity payment increases each year either in line with inflation or a suitable nominated rate. A third option is guarantee periods where the annuity is guaranteed to be paid for the remainder of the period specified. If one or both recipients die during the term, the annuity is paid to the estate.

The amount paid by annuities is determined by actuaries who take into account the amount available to purchase the annuity, age and sex of the person, current long term interest rates and life expectancy tables.

In a low interest environment, annuities are not popular as the annuity is fixed to current interest rate and provide no flexibility if additional funds are required. However, in a period of interest rates around 6-8 percent, annuities can be popular providing a stable income for the term selected.

Peer-to-peer lending (P2P lending)

Simply, peer-to-peer lending matches people or companies who have money to invest with people who are looking for a loan. Investors find borrowers through a financial service provider's online platform or website rather than going through traditional lenders such as banks, building societies or credit unions. Fees are paid by both the borrower and lender to the provider. Peer-to-peer lending platforms are set up as managed investment schemes and operators need to have an Australian Financial Services licence.

There can be many variations between lending platforms ranging from interest rates, how interest is calculated, a single loan investment or a portfolio of loans. The investor's capital may be repaid at the end of the loan period or as part of the repayments. The provider will undertake credit checks and evaluate the suitability of the borrower.

The level of risk is reflected in the comparatively high returns and there are no governed guarantees associated with funds invested in peer-to-peer lending.

Always read the Product Disclosure Statement (PDS) prior to lending any funds.

There is also other unregulated P2P lending through membership sites for property investors where people will seek loans for deposits or construction/development projects, sometimes as joint ventures or just as loans. The additional risk level here is often not reflected in the interest rates nor security offered.

P2P lending may be a relatively new term but the concept is not new. In the past, solicitors would arrange such lending between their clients.

Managed funds

In managed funds, your money is pooled with those of other investors and the investment or fund manager uses the funds to buy and sell shares or other assets on behalf of the fund. Income or distributions are paid periodically and the value of your investment in the fund rises and falls in line with the underlying assets of the fund.

Managed funds can be classed as either passive investments (index funds) where the fund portfolio mimics that of an index such as the All Ordinaries index, or it can be an actively managed fund where the fund manager aims to outperform the market by buying and selling securities.

Managed funds can be expensive and there is no guarantee of outperforming the market. They do offer diversification, allow regular contributions to be made, and provide access to a broad range of assets and markets for a relatively small investment. Unfortunately, they are not easy to liquidate if you need your funds for other purposes.

Real estate

Australians have long had a love affair with property, particularly residential property. Property has proven to be a predictable performer over a long period of time although it is not without some periods of correction; for example, the Sydney and Melbourne residential markets in 2018 and the Perth market earlier. People like the degree of control they have over property and they like the leverage – the small deposit compared to what they can borrow. Not surprisingly, the wealth of many Australians is in their family home and possibly an investment property. Despite what some politicians would have us believe, most property investors only have one investment property and the percentage of those with three or more is very small.

In the last decade, particularly in cities such as Sydney and Melbourne, the value of the family home is likely to have increased dramatically, with many now over $1 million. It is not surprising then that in the lead-up to retirement, or in retirement, the family home is considered for disposal or as an asset for a reverse mortgage. Retirees and potential retirees think of downsizing the family home, often because it is too large for just the two of them but sometimes because of financial considerations. Downsizing may be a lifestyle choice – moving to a small house at the beach or in the country or maybe a retirement village. Downsizing may also be a financial choice as a means of releasing the equity to fund retirement.

Before any decisions are made, it is important to remember some of the financial benefits of the family home. Providing the house has not been rented out, it is likely to be CGT free when you sell. Your Principal Place of Residence (PPR) is not subject to land tax and, if you are seeking a pension, the value of the home is not included in the asset test so it does not result in a reduction in the age pension. This latter point has caused retirees concern in that they have a house worth, say, $2.5 million in the inner west of Sydney but if they sell then their pension entitlements may be reduced. Many live in their house for as long as they can, survive on the pension and look at their house as a major part of their children's inheritance.

From 1 July 2018, the Australian Government has introduced what is known as 'downsizer contributions'. This allows a person over 65 years of age to contribute to their superannuation the proceeds from the sale of their principal place of residence – up to $300,000. There are a few requirements for eligibility: the house must have been owned for at least 10 years (full or partial CGT main residence exemption applies to disposal), the contribution is made within 90 days of settlement, and the approved form is used.

With residential property investment, an unemotional review needs to be carried out to determine if it will meet retirement needs. It is unlikely that negatively-geared property will have any benefit in retirement so the decision needs to be made to sell or retain. If the decision is to retain, what is the property's potential for an increase in capital growth and an increase in the rent? Is there the possibility of turning it into Airbnb, adding a granny flat, or a small boarding house? You need to check with the local council to see what may be allowed and then do an appraisal to make sure that it is worth doing. Also check with your insurance company as they may consider your property to be a commercial property.

There is also a current trend to rent houses and apartments and then sub-let these, at a higher rent, to short-term tenants through Airbnb or to the executive market. This is more common in capital cities like Sydney and Melbourne, Brisbane and Perth where there is a market with executives requiring short-term accommodation rather than hotel accommodation. While the economy is buoyant, such leasing and subleasing is fine but if there is a downturn, as Perth has experienced, then a person could have leased a property and is unable to sub-lease it.

The other option for real estate is commercial property. In recent years, commercial property has become a popular investment for SMSFs. Compared with maybe 3-4 per cent gross for residential property, commercial property is around the 6-8 per cent nett. Commercial properties generally have longer leases and the tenant pays most of the outgoings such as rates, insurance and repairs/maintenance, depending upon the terms of the lease. For a more detailed discussion on commercial property, please refer to our book *It's My Time: Introducing Commercial Investing*.

Some people like to boast about how many properties they have. The question that should be asked of these people is how much passive income they receive from these properties and whether there is any capital growth. A person with twenty properties in regional or outback Australia may receive an income but capital growth is unlikely. A person owning one or two good quality commercial properties in a major city for example, is likely to get both income and capital growth. Owning many properties and having to deal with different property managers and tenant requests for maintenance may not be the type of retirement you have contemplated.

Shares

Shares are another asset class that many Australians are familiar with. In fact, Australia has one of the highest ownerships of shares in the world. Most working Australians will have exposure to shares through their superannuation fund or may have directly purchased shares. Those who are a little older may have acquired shares in the Commonwealth Bank or Telstra when they became publicly listed companies rather than government-owned institutions.

The value of shares is primarily determined by the type of business and how well it operates. For example the Commonwealth Bank is held in higher regard than Telstra and this is reflected in the share price. The Australian share price can be influenced by what happens overseas and it is not uncommon for a drop on the Wall Street exchange to adversely affect the Australian share market the next day.

At other times, a company may decide to issue more shares, sometimes as bonus shares, and this can affect the share price. If one of our banks was trading at $60 per share, and decided to issue each shareholder with 100 shares for each share that they hold on a particular date, then by issuing these additional shares the share price has been diluted and the price drops to $0.60 per share.

Shares are easy to purchase through a full-service stockbroker or an online broker. A relatively small amount of capital is required to purchase shares. Brokerage or commission is charged for buying and selling shares and can be a percentage rate or a flat fee. Australians can purchase shares listed on the Australian Stock Exchange or shares listed on many International stock exchanges. There are a number of different ways to classify shares… Firstly, there are Australian shares and international shares, depending upon which stock exchange the shares are listed on. Next, we can have speculative and non-speculative shares, the main difference being the risk involved and the underlying assets of the company. A speculative share could be associated with a new start-up company, for example a mining company or, in days gone by, tech stocks. Non-speculative stocks are shares of major Australian companies.

Non-speculative shares can be classified a number of ways, two of which are as preference shares and ordinary shares. Both shares are similar except that preference shares have a different dividend payment arrangement and, if the company was wound up, they have a preferred position in the distribution of any assets of the company. The dividend rate for preference shares is set at the issue date and these dividends are given priority over ordinary shares in the payment of any dividend.

Another terminology common to describe non-speculative shares is 'blue chip'. These are companies that have substantial assets, are well known and generally have a long history of paying dividends. Examples are the major four Australian banks, BHP and Woolworths. The prices for non-speculative shares are not as volatile as the speculative shares and dividends are more likely to be paid.

Many of these blue chip companies pay a fully-franked dividend if the company operates in Australia and pays taxes in Australia. Some companies also operate outside of Australia and pay tax overseas so only issue a partially-franked dividend based on the proportion of the tax paid in Australia. Franking or imputation credits were introduced to stop double taxation. The company pays tax at 30 cents in the dollar profit and then distributes some or all of that profit to shareholders as dividends. The shareholders would then include that dividend in their tax return and pay tax on that dividend. The franking credit allows the shareholder to offset the proportion of the amount of tax that the company has paid against any tax the shareholder has to pay. In the case of retirees who may pay no tax, they receive a cash refund from the Australian Taxation Office.

The proposed changes to franking dividends for pensioners, which would have meant that the retirees would not receive this cash refund, was one factor that was attributed to Labour losing the 'unlosable' election in 2019.

Speculative stocks can also include shares termed 'penny dreadfuls' which are stocks in a company that has little asset backing, may have a new innovation or own the exploration rights over a particular area; the shares are purchased on the prospect of the company becoming successful. There is a prospect of large profits for a relatively small outlay or, if the company goes into liquidation, a total loss. The penny dreadfuls price can also be influenced by unfounded rumours of success so the price can fluctuate wildly. Some companies also issue options giving the owner of these options the right to buy or sell a particular share at a particular price on a particular day in the future. Options can be traded on the stock exchange like their parent company. They are inexpensive to purchase but they are risky, particularly as their expiry date draws nearer.

Other sources of income

Unlike our parents or grandparents whose retirement income was the age or invalid pension, or a war service pension, there are a number of other ways that retirees can supplement their income.

Older Australians are twice as likely to be self-employed than younger Australians. This may occur as a result of a long-held passion to undertake some venture, turning a hobby into a business, or a desire to help offspring into their own business. The older person brings experience, connections and generally financial resources to the business. So what are some of the ventures that people may consider?

Turning interests or hobbies into a business

Any hobby may be a potential source of income in retirement. Carpentry expertise could produce all types of wooden products from doll houses, children's furniture and toys to hand made tables and chairs. Do you have a talent with a paintbrush or a camera? Does your hobby have the potential to earn you money? Do you like gardening and maybe propagating plants? Do any friends grow their own vegetables or herbs? Is there a possibility of swapping some of your home-grown vegetables for some of their vegetables? Do you grow any Asian vegetables that a local Thai, Indian or Chinese takeaway might be interested in purchasing?

Do you have some computer skills, writing skills or other abilities that may be marketable through companies like Fiverr?

Taxation Services

There are a number of companies providing taxation services that seek additional staff during the busy tax season from July to November. You would be required to undertake a tax training course over approximately 16 weeks at a cost of about $500. You would need a Windows compatible computer, a printer and internet access. If you are offered a job as a tax consultant after completing the course, you will be paid at an hourly casual rate, and possibly overtime and superannuation.

Writing / Proofreading

Have you thought of writing a book – children's, fiction or non-fiction or perhaps a blog such as a travel blog of your trips either overseas or around Australia? Do you have a good understanding of the English language and could you proofread manuscripts? Look at websites like Fiverr and Freelancer for work for your particular skills.

Competitions and Jingles

Whilst it may not be considered income, some people can reduce their expenditure by entering competitions. Prizes can vary considerably from a product only worth a few dollars to overseas trips or in one case that we know of, a new kitchen. A number of years ago, a tax client of mine made some handy pocket money from writing jingles.

Market Research

There are a number of companies that seek people to review food and drinks as well as other products. As well as earning some money, it provides a chance to meet new people.

Online Selling

There are many other new and interesting ways of earning money both in the lead-up to and in retirement. Through the likes of Amazon and Ebay, people are buying and selling products online. Others are buying websites to renovate and sell.

In recent years, we have seen a number of new ways to earn an income with little capital outlay, flexible hours and working from home. We will look at a few of the more popular examples…

Ride sharing

We will use Uber as an example for this category of income but bear in mind that there are now a number of new players such as *Didi* and *Ola*. The attraction with ride sharing is that it can be full-time or part-time and, being your own boss you are able to set the hours that you want to work. There are minimal requirements to commence – a vehicle in good condition (normally less than 10 years old), insured and roadworthy. The driver must have a full driver's licence and a passport so that a background check can be undertaken. Apart from the income from fares, there are some discount fuel and mobile phone plans and a few other benefits available; for example, bonuses which may be based on having performed a certain number of trips in a day.

There may be other requirements and costs depending upon the state or territory where the rideshare operates.

Homestay accommodation (Airbnb and StayZ)

Because we have briefly mentioned Airbnb previously, we will refer to Airbnb here in regard to other homestay accommodation.

Airbnb is an online platform connecting people who want to rent out a room, boat, caravan or other property to people looking for accommodation in a particular area. Airbnb is in more than 81,000 cities and towns in some 191 countries around the world.

It is relatively simple to list a property on Airbnb. Whether renting a room or an entire house, declutter and clean the area before getting professional photographs taken. Check to see what your competition is in the area and how it compares so that you have an idea of price. Write the advertisement highlighting any unique features, amenities and closeness to public transport. Check with the local council, strata manager if applicable, and the insurance company to ensure there are no issues with renting through Airbnb. Airbnb charges hosts a 3 per cent payment processing fee and the guests are charged between 6 and 12 per cent as a booking fee.

Airbnb is relatively new in Australia. State and local governments are still coming to terms with how to treat homestay accommodation although they do have experience with traditional bed and breakfast accommodation. In many areas in Australia, Airbnb is unregulated and causing angst with many locals. So what could we expect of regulators if overseas experience is any indication…?

In Japan, laws from 2018 require hosts to obtain a licence placing a 180-day quota on renting properties and shutting down those properties that did not comply. Airbnb reportedly has been fined over $10 million.

Berlin laws ban short-term leasing of properties to tourists without a city permit and hosts who disobey this law can face fines up to €100,000.

Paris is planning to follow Berlin and increase fines for hosts from €25,000 to €100,000. Hosts are required to obtain a registration number from the town hall to make it easier to monitor the 120-day cap and ensure taxes are paid.

Barcelona has reportedly fined Airbnb €600,000 for refusing to adhere to local laws by continuing to advertise unlicensed properties. New fines of €60,000 for hosts are being introduced.

San Francisco has implemented a 90-day cap on entire home listings and owners can be fined for renting without a permit. Platforms like Airbnb face fines of $1,000 per day for illegal listings.

New York local laws make it illegal to rent an entire apartment on Airbnb for less than 30 days. This is aimed at helping to maintain the long-term supply of property available to locals.

In Jersey City, an ordinance passed in June establishes a 60-day annual cap on short-term rental properties if the owner is not on site. It prohibits Airbnb rentals in buildings with more than four units. It will also phase out existing short-term rental contracts by 1 January 2021 and prohibit renters from serving as short-term hosts.

Some overseas cities impose a bed or occupancy tax on home rentals. For example, Massachusetts has a 5.7 per cent excise tax for rentals of more than $15 per day and Boston 6.5 per cent.

Australia has been slow to adjust to Airbnb and some of the experiences in overseas cities seem likely to be introduced in some Australian cities and towns. Airbnb appears to be dividing some smaller communities and councils are starting to take action with bylaws to regulate Airbnb properties.

Airbnb has moved from mums and dads renting out space in their homes for a modest profit to entire homes and apartments being rented out. Promoters have new courses on Airbnb, encouraging multiple listings of properties by a single host. Promoters are encouraging people to lease a property on a long-term basis and then subletting it to sub-tenants for short-term stays charging up to 300 per cent of the long-term rental paid.

In Victoria, the owner of an apartment took the tenants to the Victoria Civil and Administrative Tribunal (VCAT) when the owner discovered the apartment was being sublet unlawfully to a third party. VCAT ruled that the tenants had not sublet. The owner then took the case to the Supreme Court which overturned the VCAT ruling. The sublease was considered a breach of the tenant's lease which prohibited subleasing.

The Australian Taxation Office (ATO) has recently given notice to Airbnb to provide information regarding hosting activities for the period 2016-2020. The ATO argues that the sharing economy lets people operate commercial arrangements which can be used to evade tax including CGT and GST. It is possible that the current crackdown announced by the ATO might be the tip of the iceberg if they then start to look at CGT and GST. Some promoters of Airbnb schemes report incomes of over $200,000 per year so well above the GST threshold. Residential rentals are not subject to GST so we will have to watch as this unfolds.

Councils and various government departments may also start looking at safety regulations, fire and disability access regulations. Some recent high-rise apartment crises in Sydney and Melbourne have also highlighted issues with Airbnb rentals greatly increasing the number of residents in such buildings. One private certifier has said that if he had known that the building would be used for Airbnb, he would have classified the building differently.

The Australian Building Codes Board (ABCB) released a discussion paper *The National Construction Code and Short Term Accommodation in Apartment Buildings in March 2018.*

International students

If you have a spare bedroom and your house is within a reasonable distance of a university and good public transport then there is potential for extra income by hosting international students. It is also a chance to learn about different cultures. As well as providing a bedroom, you are also required to provide meals and maybe some transport.

Some universities that run English language classes for overseas students may have a department within the university which manages home stays. There are also private providers that organise homestays for overseas students.

Our experience with homestay students has been very positive. We have had students stay with us for a few days but one student who initially came for five weeks stayed for more than two years. It can be a very rewarding way to make use of the large family home. Not only financially, but with friendships that can develop. Our students to date have come from Colombia, Japan, China, Timor Lestre, Italy, Taiwan and South Korea; and we still remain in contact with a number of them.

Investment risks

All investments come with a risk. Even leaving money in the bank for a long term has inherent risks. We will take a look at a number of these risks so that you are aware of them…

For retirees, a major risk is inflation; particularly for those with a defensive investment strategy. As the price of goods and services increases through inflation, the purchasing power for retirees decreases because their income remains the same. This is relevant if invested primarily in income-producing investments with little or no capital growth. This is the major problem for money left in the bank for a long term.

There is also the risk associated with interest rates. Will housing interest rates fall further and when should the interest rate be fixed on a home loan? Similarly, if money is invested in a bank deposit, should it be fixed? Currently in Australia, interest rates are at an all-time low level both for earnings on any deposits and also for home loan interest rates. At some stage, interest rates will increase. Those that have locked in term deposits may then lose as the interest rates climb above what they are receiving on their money. It can also work against borrowers. Borrowers that lock in interest rates at 8 per cent for a 5 year fixed term and then find interest rates drop to 3-4 per cent over the next eighteen months, are at a disadvantage. (But note that they will have been at an advantage for the period that the variable rates were above 8 per cent). They are likely to incur penalties to change to a lower interest rate before the fixed term expires.

For many older retirees and those with a significant property portfolio, liquidity risk can be a real fear. This is the fear of running out of money. It can be a real fear for many retirees – outliving the nest egg that has been built up over a lifetime. Fortunately, there is the age pension to fall back on. Also for those with a significant part of their SMSF tied up in property, liquidity risk can be a major issue when it comes to meeting the requirements to pay the minimum pension as required by law.

Other risks are associated with markets and market timing. Any products bought or sold in a market-place such as shares, property or cryptocurrencies are subject to these two risks. As markets are governed by emotion and sentiment rather than facts and logic, markets can rise and fall sometimes quite wildly. This has happened in the dot.com bubble, the property crashes in mining towns like Moranbah and Port Hedland, and in 2018 with Bitcoin. It may also happen over a period of time such as housing in Sydney and Melbourne and the drop in prices during 2018 and early 2019. The second part of the risk involves market timing where people predict that the market will continue to rise or, for some, when it will fall. People have listened to overseas and home-grown experts and sold their shares or property based on a predicted crash or depression. Nobody can predict the market or market timing accurately.

We have all heard about not having all your eggs in the one basket and diversification. Generally this is sound advice but there are risks associated with diversification as well as concentration. We know the risk of not diversifying and having our investments concentrated in one class of investment or one investment in a class of investments; fluctuations within that class or the one investment can seriously affect the value of your portfolio. But there are also dangers with having too broad a diversification both in the cost of administration and in keeping abreast of changes in the various investments.

For those with investments overseas such as in New Zealand or the USA, currency risk is a major consideration. The risk is associated with the movement of the Australian dollar in relationship to the overseas currency that the investment is held in. For example, a property investment in the USA may require additional funds to be sent to the USA to meet a large unexpected expense or a property has been sold and you wish to transfer funds back to Australia. If you have time then you may be able to wait for a more favourable exchange rate but often this is not the case. There are also various bank fees associated with the transfers.

For some more sophisticated investors, they may go into joint venture arrangements as money partners or lend money to private lenders and this makes them subject to a credit risk. This is where the borrower defaults on the money lent and you lose not only the funds but interest at the rate that was promised.

There are also risks associated with policy and taxation changes by the various levels of government. The Federal Government appears to tinker with superannuation with each budget announcement and, in the lead-up to the 2019 Federal election, Labour was proposing changes to negative gearing. What changes may happen in the future to health care or pensions? The age of being able to access the pension is gradually increasing. Again, if you have overseas investments, your investments may be subject to changes by the overseas government.

We also face event risks which may be an economic event such as a global financial crisis (GFC), a depression or a more personal event such as major renovations being required to your house to allow for wheelchair access.

The final two risks are health-related. Firstly, there is the risk associated with declining health as we age and how that may affect us financially. Secondly, there is the risk of increased longevity causing a shortfall of funds. On the other hand, you may have taken out a lifetime pension and you live for less time than you expected.

Do you have a risk management plan? How much can you afford to lose without endangering your lifestyle? Where do you intend to take risk and what is the percentage of this risk against the total sum of these risks? There is always a risk/return trade-off so, over the longer term, the less risk you take the lower the return is expected.

Your attitude to risk will, and should, influence your investment portfolio.

How can risk be managed?

Investment risk can be managed in a number of ways…

1 The length of time that an investment is held lowers the risk of it falling in value. There is an old saying, 'it is the time in the market that makes money, not trying to time the markets'. Time is your friend.

2 Your risk tolerance is influenced by age so it is important to review your portfolio regularly. Consider setting percentage limits for each investment across investment classes. Limit your exposure to volatile assets

3 Diversify the investment portfolio across investment classes like cash, fixed interest, residential property, commercial property, Australian shares and international shares

4 Sensible tax planning is important but it should never be the prime motivation for any investment decision

5 Is there a way of transferring risk? For example, the risk of exhausting capital before dying may be offset by an indexed lifetime annuity

6 Listen to your own intuition or gut feelings. Don't follow the herd into investments and weigh up all advice. If it sounds too good to be true, it probably is – so start running.

Government benefits available

There are a number of commonwealth and state government benefits available to people who meet various eligibility requirements.

The Commonwealth Seniors Health Card is issued to people who have reached age pension age with a taxable income of less than $55,808 for singles and $89,290 for couples or $111,616 for couples separated by illness. (taxable income as at 20 September 2020) There is no asset test applicable for this health card.

There is also the Pensioner Concession Card which is issued to anyone receiving a pension, carer payment or parenting payment. This card provides the same medical concessions as the Health Care Card plus access to rebates on various utilities like water, energy and rates.

State Government Seniors Card

Once you turn 60 in all states apart from cheapskate Queensland, you are entitled to a variety of concessions providing you meet the eligibility tests such as the number of hours worked. The concessions available, range from reduced fares on public transport to reduction in motor vehicle registration and varies from state to state.

Reassessing your investments

Not all investments may have turned out to be as great as the salesperson had us believe. Now is the time to have a good look at what investments are held and critically evaluate whether those assets that have not performed should be kept going into retirement or changed to another fund manager or maybe it is time to bite the bullet and dispose of them?

This evaluation should cover all assets such as shares, property, superannuation or other 'investments' like wine, gold, coins or other collectables.

We had to face this reality with a wine collection that we started to accumulate in 2005. We had wine stored in Sydney and in the United Kingdom and the history of wine sales, at the time of purchase, had indicated that we should realise a profit when we came to sell. Unfortunately the GFC had an adverse effect on people buying good wines but also the company storing the wine changed hands with a management buyout. New charges were introduced, the service diminished and, for some unknown reasons, they changed storage locations both in Sydney and in the United Kingdom – all at the investor's expense.

For the last three years we have been attempting to sell our wine and at least 90 percent of the wine that we have sold to date has been at a significant loss after all the fees and charges were taken into account.

There are a couple of lessons that we have learned from this 'investment'. Firstly, you must understand your investment and the market. Secondly, when the management buyout occurred and the new charges started to appear, we should have either moved our wine to a new storage facility and new selling agent, or immediately started to dispose of the wine. We may still have suffered a loss on the sale but would have saved thousands of dollars in storage fees. Thirdly, it takes far longer to dispose of an asset than you might think. Lastly, there is no benefit in taking losses into retirement if you are not going to have a taxable income to offset them against.

Similarly, there is no such investment as a set-and-forget. Some investments will require less management but there are none that you can forget. Make it a point to review all your investments and your investment plan regularly because situations change, investment returns change and you need to be aware of these changes and how they affect your investment strategy.

Controlling expenditure

Regardless of your previous lifestyle, preparing for retirement is going to necessitate a review of expenditure both now and into the future. For people that have been thrifty during their working life, things may not change much but for people who have enjoyed a good lifestyle, then things may have to change. Remember the old saying 'a leopard can't change its spots'; so those who have enjoyed a good lifestyle may have to work hard to change.

In retirement, it is more important than ever to live within our means whilst allowing for daily expenses that make life worth living; and now is the time to start. It is important not to cut anything out of your spending until you know that it is necessary to do so or you are certain that it will not be required in your new life. The unfortunate reality is that you will need to allow for increasing health costs or preventative costs like gym fees as you age.

Unfortunately, some people can become mentally paralysed once they lose a regular income. Before retirement they may have looked forward to an overseas holiday, comfortable in the knowledge that they would be going back to work and would have an income coming in to pay for the expenses that may have gone onto the credit card.

However, a retired person may feel very uncomfortable taking a similar overseas holiday just after they have retired, concerned that there is no pay packet to return to.

For many retirees entering retirement, having a bank balance equal to at least six months of income that can then be progressively drawn down each fortnight or month may provide some peace of mind in the initial retirement months.

Pre-retirement is the time to commence getting debts and expenses under control and practise taking an overseas holiday, assuming no salary or wage to come back to.

Debts

If you have debts, whether in the form of mortgages, personal loans, car loans or credit cards, now is the time to consider how you are going to repay these loans. Some people are happy to have a mortgage as a form of asset protection but this strategy needs to be discussed by all parties to see if it is appropriate and everyone is comfortable with such a strategy. Some reduction of debt to a manageable level may need to be considered?

There is one school of thought that a loan principal should not be repaid but left to the estate for finalisation but this may not be the appropriate action to take. Loan repayments can be a cause of financial stress and this will be heightened if there is no regular income from salary and wages to meet the loan repayments. Also, loans normally have a term attached to them, whether it is a

30 year principal and interest loan or a fixed 5 year interest only loan, so there will be a time at which the banks will be looking for the loan to be repaid.

Start with the loan with the highest interest rate and work out a plan to pay down that loan as quickly as possible. Once this loan is paid down, select the next highest interest rate loan and repeat. If you receive any bonuses or other lump sums, use those to make a lump sum payment on the loan. If you receive a pay increase then don't increase your living expenses. Keep your living expenses the same and put that extra money from the pay increase to paying down the loan. Similarly, if there is a reduction in your interest rate on a loan, then keep your repayments the same as they were with the higher rate and that will also help to reduce your loan balance.

It is also worth making a phone call to your bank and asking what the best interest rate is that they can offer. We recently made such a phone call and were offered a reduction of 0.88 per cent on our loan, a saving in excess of $6,000 per annum. Such a saving will also assist in any debt reduction strategy.

Be sensible about debt. Be comfortable with the debt that you have and that you can afford it in retirement whilst still being able to enjoy a comfortable lifestyle.

Insurances

Now is a good time to review your insurance needs. If you own a car and a house then car insurance and house/contents insurances are a must have. It is important that you are comfortable with the amount you have them insured for, particularly your house. You don't want your house to be underinsured so it is important that you get a good idea of what the replacement cost would be if your house was destroyed by fire or a natural disaster. There are a number of calculators on various websites that can assist you in calculating a replacement cost for your house.

Have you compared your current policy and premiums with others in the market-place? Too often, the renewal notice arrives via email or in the post and is automatically paid without any comparison. Compare it with others; are there items that are no longer required to be covered or are there new items to be added? Can you get a discount by having multiple policies with the same insurer? Is there a seniors discount applicable? Ask the questions – you may be surprised by the result.

Health insurance is another that you need to keep but ensure that you review what is covered. Pregnancy costs may not be required for a 65 year old female but it may be part of your current package if you have not reviewed your health insurance for some time. It is also important to find out what benefits the health insurer may provide in terms of keeping fit; for example gym membership or a pilates course. One day, health insurers will come to realise that if they are serious about health then they should be providing more benefits toward keeping people fit and thereby having less claims for costly medical procedures.

There are two types of life insurance – a whole of life and term life. The whole of life insurance has a life insurance as well as an investment component which is payable on your death but also if you reach a certain age. It has been a costly insurance so most life insurance sold over the last 30 plus years has been term life. It is the insurance that is attached to most superannuation policies or the one that the banks had you take out when you applied for a home loan. It is relatively cheap and is designed to protect your family in the event of your death by paying out large debts like your home loan or investment loan. It was never intended to provide a nest egg for your family's future happiness.

If you have been paying down your home and investment loans through principal and interest loans then it would be prudent to review your life insurance and decide whether it is still relevant. If you have a SMSF then a review of your life insurance is one thing that should be undertaken annually.

Life insurance gets more expensive as you get older, so if you are looking at some cost savings as you enter retirement, then review your insurances. This may be important if you have a superannuation fund through your employer as it is likely to have a life insurance component.

If you have Total and Permanent Disability insurance (TPD) and or Income Protection Insurance (IPI), you may question whether you still require this insurance if you are going to retire in the next year or two. If you were to make a claim, over what period would the insurance company pay you? Some insurance companies will only pay monthly benefits until you reach age 60 or 65 – so is it worth the premium?

If, however, your retirement is 5, 10 or more years away, then life insurance and income protection income should be considered as an important part of risk management in planning retirement. A serious accident or illness can have a major impact on preparing for your retirement.

Finance allocation

Interestingly, we have been told to save for our retirement but the majority of us have no idea of what our retirement journey is going to be like. Do you have an inspirational vision of what you would do if you were financially able, money being no object?

For most of us, we will have to consider our spending as our income may be limited by our investment income or part-time work. Some simple adjustments now can create large improvements in all areas such as finance and health.

One important thing to consider is the allocation of your income and categorising your expenses.

You may have heard of *Maslow's Hierarchy of Needs*. You can develop a similar hierarchy to allocate your income. We suggest six categories in our hierarchy of needs but you may have fewer.

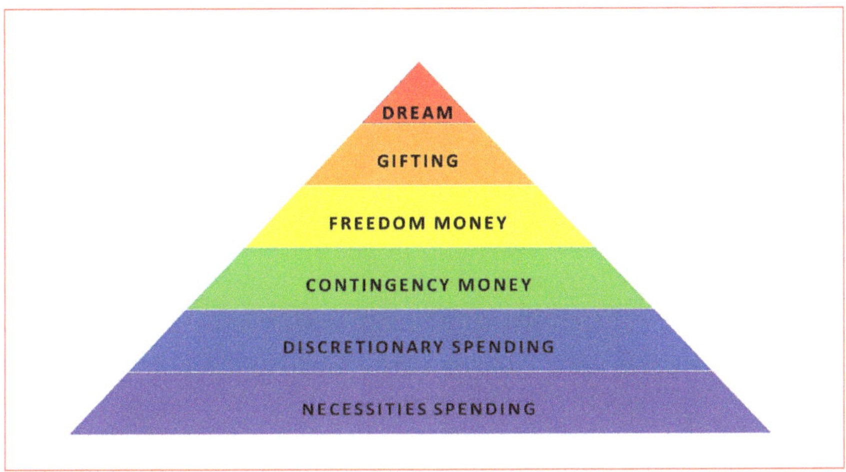

At the base of the triangle there are necessities or essentials, the funds that you need for your survival. This covers basic food and clothing, shelter, medical needs and transportation for your day-to-day living. The expenses included in this category will depend on the individual as basic needs will vary greatly.

The second level is discretionary spending which relates to your lifestyle choices. Entertainment, alcohol, donations and holidays are some examples of what may be included. They are not the necessities for living but provide some pleasure.

The next level up is security or contingency money. The contingency reserve is where you build up a nest-egg to meet unexpected expenses or emergencies. The amount that you feel you need in this reserve, will depend to some extent on your risk profile. This will cover expenditure that may be unforeseen like major car repairs or house repairs, serious illness or death in the family, loss of a job or a once-off major expenditure like replacing a car. Each person will have a different risk tolerance; those with a low risk tolerance may allocate more to their security money. If you are concerned that you may outlive your retirement funds, you may want to put more into this security bucket.

The next level is your play or freedom money where you allocate funds to cover things that you enjoy to do and which bring joy to your life. It could be hobbies, travel, learning a language or some other intellectual pursuit, membership of golf/tennis clubs or fitness gyms or maybe owning a boat, caravan and a 4WD fitted out for touring.

One level from the pinnacle is gifting or charitable giving. Are there particular causes or charities that you want to support? Do you want to help with a grandchild's education or help them get into their first home? Would you like to establish a scholarship fund or donate to a school or university? Maybe there is a close friend or even a stranger that you have heard is having a tough time and you can help. In Australia, there are always appeals to help victims of floods, bushfires, cyclones and drought.

The pinnacle of your pyramid is your dream money. What do you dream of owning – boat, plane, vintage car or motorbike? Are there places that you dream of going to such as travelling around Australia or maybe around the world? What are your dreams?

The aim of this book is to examine a holistic retirement plan. We have attempted to keep this chapter brief, touching on areas without going into depth but, as you have seen, there are many things that need to be considered in the lead-up to retirement, particularly in regards to your financial planning.

Three final remarks:

Most people will tend to significantly under-estimate their retirement income needs so think carefully about your future lifestyle and do not under-estimate the expenditure or over-estimate the income.

Procrastination has never, and will never, be a sensible strategy for retirement planning so start now.

As well as financially, we need to prepare ourselves physically and mentally for leaving work.

Financial aspects to consider

Expenses	Current expenditure	Estimated post-retirement expenditure	Comments
	Expenditure		
Food			
Alcohol			
Clothing			
Dry cleaning			
Hairdressing			
Electricity			
Rates and water			
House and contents insurance			
Telephone			
Internet			
Cleaning			
Repairs and home maintenance			
Mortgage			
Entertainment			
Gym membership			
Life insurance			
Income protection insurance			
Health insurance			
Car insurance			
Car maintenance			
Fuel			
Car registration			
Transport fares			
Superannuation contributions			
Memberships			
Credit card repayments			
Gifts and birthday presents			
Donations			
Other			
Total			

Assets and liabilities				
Asset	Owned by	Estimated value	Amount owed	Retain in retirement
Family Home				
Investment property 1				
Investment property 2				
Investment property 3				
Holiday home				
Superannuation				
SMSF				
Term deposits				
Shares				
Managed investments				
Cash at bank				
Other				
Motor vehicles				
Caravan				
Boat				
Motor bike				
Tools of trade				
Credit card limits		Nil		
Personal loan balance		Nil		
Total				

Key learnings from this chapter

Chapter 5

Psychology

The best time to start thinking about your retirement is before the boss does.

Author unknown

In the chapter on health, we will look at some practices that you can start now to keep your mind and body healthy in retirement. But retirement also needs to be looked at from a psychological point of view as it is a major change in your life.

In his book, *The Process of Retirement*, Robert Atchley outlines six stages in the retirement process:

1. Pre-retirement in which plans are made and attitudes about retirement are formed
2. Retirement day, often marked by celebration – but not always
3. Honeymoon period which ranges from a few months to a year where people are relaxed and happy with no daily structure and less stress. It is sometimes seen as an extended holiday.
4. Disenchantment is a time during which people feel a lack of purpose, lost and confused but knowing that they need new life goals and to develop a routine. Too long in this phase can lead to feeling trapped and depressed.
5. Reorientation is where people start to adjust to a retirement lifestyle, their attitude and behaviour change to cope more effectively
6. Routine is established that meets their personal and marital needs.

Thankfully, there is now no mandatory retirement age of 65 and people now have the ability to choose when they wish to retire.

For some it may be sooner and for others much later; some have no intention of retiring.

The lead-up to retirement can be quite mixed. There may be anticipation and excitement as we near retirement, anxiety and possibly regret as we think about what we might be losing in terms of income and workmates. If married or in a partnership, it is important to discuss options and make plans together.

You must remember that retirement is not just for one day – the day that you leave work for the last time – but it is the start of an ongoing process with significant and long-lasting impact on you, the retiree, and those closest to you.

So why do people retire at different ages and what are some of the facts to consider with retirement?

Loss of employment

All of your life, you have been career or work-focused. Do you remember as a child being asked 'what are you going to be when you grow up'? Now you are grown up, but few people want to know about your next stage of life.

Your best-made plans do not always work out the way you would like and, unfortunately, you may not be able to work as long as you had hoped. This may be as a result of an accident or illness forcing you to end your work early or it may be as a result of losing your job through the company closing down or downsizing the workforce. Regardless of when this may happen in your career, it is never an easy thing to cope with financially or mentally. How you address this loss of employment as you approach retirement can have long term consequences on how you view your retirement. People who suffer loss of employment through downsizing often experience a loss of confidence and self-esteem even when they may have been expecting such an event.

Those who enjoy retirement the most have a positive mental attitude, they can handle changes that are likely to happen and, in general, have a determination to get on with life. They turn negatives into positives and are confident that they will find other work if they choose to look.

Sometimes there is the opportunity to take voluntary redundancy from your employer. Research has shown that, psychologically, you are better to take voluntary redundancy than to be made redundant. The big difference here is that you are in control and have decided you are ready to move on; to retirement, other full-time work or even part-time work.

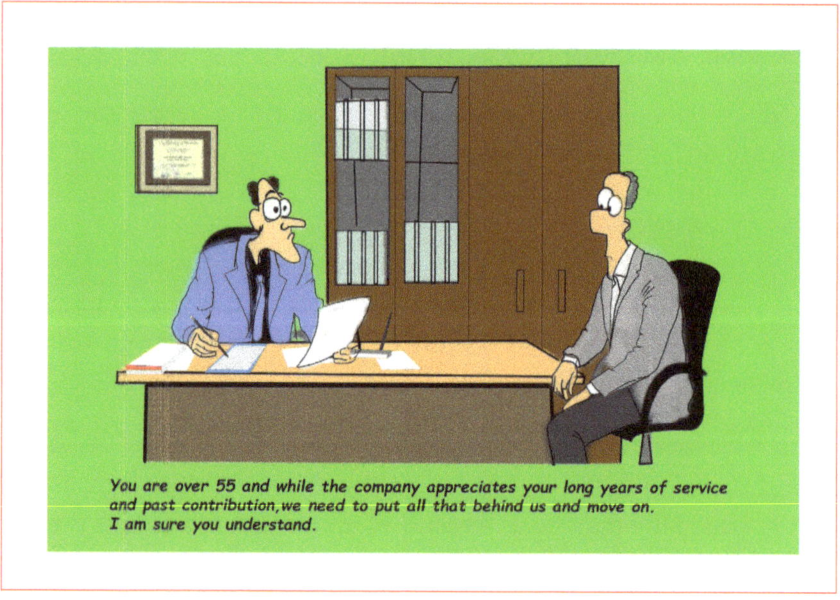

Loss of identity/ Loss of status

For many, the biggest fear in retirement comes with the loss of identity. For better or worse, in our society you are what you do. You go to parties or a function and one of the first questions by way of introduction is 'what do you do for a living?'. Many have been able to associate with a particular profession or organisation so, when asked this at a party, they can respond that they are a manager at a particular company. Seldom after you retire will you be introduced as the ex-manager or the ex-CEO for a particular company; you will just be introduced as Joe Smith and, when asked what you do, your answer may not be a topic-starter for a further conversation.

The loss of identity is particularly relevant for professionals or senior managers but it can affect anyone planning to retire in one form or another. Many people are not emotionally prepared to deal with their identity without work.

Have you considered a 'bridging' identity? Is there something that you enjoy and are good at that you could develop between now and retirement so that people will come to know you for that skill? It could be in baking, market gardening, organising social events or school fetes. What skills do you have that could be beneficial to others? It does not necessarily have to be a money-making venture.

Loss of intellectual stimulus

Most work environments provide varying degrees of intellectual stimulus. Professional and clerical workers may have more stimulus than some others but all of us are likely to suffer a loss of intellectual stimulus when we retire. Again, the transition period leading up to retirement is the time to think about what will provide an intellectual stimulus when you retire. It could be as simple as a crossword or sudoku, a puzzle or volunteer work. There is no reason for you to lose your intellectual stimulus. As well as leisure, there is a wide variety of activities that you can become involved in to provide the intellectual stimulus – commence further studies at university or learn a language, use your skills and experience as a coach or mentor, undertake part-time work, become a consultant or start a new business. We write more about this in the chapter on health. Building and maintaining intellectual stimulus also aids your self-esteem.

Loss of structure

Work also provides a structure to our lives. We had a time to be at work, a time for lunch and a time to finish our day's work. In retirement, you now need to find a meaningful replacement in order to bring structure back into your life otherwise you may spend half the day in bed. Morning walks, going to the gym or meeting a friend for an early coffee are useful activities to start the day – so why not build them into your days now?

Loss of respect

In the past, retirement was closely associated with age and with age-perceived knowledge and wisdom which led to respect. In many cultures around the world, elders within the community are highly respected.

Today, youth and vitality are often seen as more valuable. Even in the workforce, once a certain perceived age is reached, opportunities for education, training and advancement seem to pass you by. For some time there appears to have been some ill-feeling towards the Boomers by the Gen X and Gen Y who want the boomers to retire so that they can take on the managerial roles.

Perhaps Boomers have partly brought this upon themselves. Prior to the mid 1970s, anyone that was 10 or 15 years your senior was referred to as Mr Smith, Mrs Smith or Miss Smith as a sign of respect. Somewhere along the way, this disappeared and was replaced by calling people by their christian names and possibly the start of the decline.

Loss of perspective

Some people still think of retirement as having one foot in the grave. This should never be the situation and in the lead-up to retirement it is important that we don't develop that mindset. Unfortunately, we have all experienced it. A classic example is when retirees or pre-retirees purchase a new vehicle with the attitude that this vehicle will 'see them out'. With such an attitude, it is likely that the vehicle will last longer than they will. People in their forties or fifties are unlikely to make such a comment so why should people in their sixties or seventies?

Loss of purpose

Work provides many people with a purpose in life. They may get recognition for the work they have done but they also have a sense of pride in the work that they do as well as knowing that they are providing financially for their family. What do you need to do to feel productive, worthwhile and valuable without the job that has been your life for so many years?

Feeling industrious is almost a prerequisite for success in retirement.

How do you view retirement?

Is it a time for a well-earned holiday, more time to spend with family and friends, a time to develop new skills or reactivate ones that you have not had time for? Is there going to be a lot of travel or volunteer work? At least one third of retirees experience difficulties with the transition to retirement.

Don't compare yourself with others

We all go through life comparing ourselves, whether consciously or not, with other people. We do not have to do it, particularly as we head for retirement. There is no real expectation of what a retiree should be like so why try to compare ourselves with anyone else? Men, if you want to swap your suit for a hippy lifestyle, grow a beard and shoulder length hair, who cares? (Apart from your spouse, that is).

Whether rich or poor, whether you live in a mansion or a shack near the beach, it is just your perception that others may be looking up to you or frowning at you.

Today, retirement expectations are much higher than our parents' generation. Baby Boomers want, and expect, more of retirement as they are generally physically and financially better off. But not everyone wants the same thing.

You are now entering a phase of your life when you can be who you want to be – so think about it and enjoy it.

Imagine one less thing that you have to worry about in life.

What to do with 'free time'

As some people with parents who have been retired for a while will know, there does not seem to be a lot of free time. Often we were told by both parents and parents-in-law when we tried to arrange an outing or a get-together, 'we will need to check our diary'. The idea that retirees do nothing but sit in a rocking chair waiting for the pearly gates to open is far from reality.

It is good to be occupied and it is important to carefully consider the use of your time. If you are grandparents, it is also important to place some constraints on the times that you may be available to babysit or pick up children from school. It is good to be able to help your children and you may enjoy spending time with your grandchildren but remember that you have a life to live as well. Now is the time to start those 1001 things you have always wanted to do but never had the time.

Time is the most valuable commodity that you have, particularly as you get older, so it is important to make the best use of your time. The question of what is the best use of a person's time will depend on the individual.

Loneliness

We are not talking here of people who chose to live alone because people who live alone are not necessarily lonely. Loneliness can affect people living in families as well as a single person. Loneliness is a major concern as we plan and enter into retirement. Unfortunately, death, divorce and potentially loss of a job can all lead to loneliness. Loneliness can have major implications for our health and finances. It means that people may withdraw, not eat properly, not exercise and, if they do go out, it may be to the casino or local club to play the pokies. Gambling and loneliness can be a major detriment to our finances. Loneliness can be bad for both our physical and mental health, heightening our risk of death. Research has shown that lonely people feel more anxious and report feelings of low self-esteem.

People living on their own should find a balance between solitary pursuits and social activities. It is important to arrange a regular weekly or monthly get-together with friends rather than texting or a phone call. Joining a gym and going regularly to meet your gym buddies is great. Always keep an eye on how much alcohol you drink while out of the house but particularly when alone at home.

If there are no close children or siblings, you may have growing concerns as you get older about who may take care of you when your health fails.

Maybe not surprisingly, men are most at risk of loneliness particularly when widowed or divorced. Their partners have normally been the ones to make sure that they ate correctly, exercised and undertook jobs around the house and pushed them to see a doctor if feeling unwell. So men generally have problems looking after themselves unless they have had extended periods where they have had to look after themselves in the past.

Loneliness is a major 'disease' and the more that it is identified and steps put in place to control it, the happier and healthier everyone will be.

When will I know it is time to retire?

This is a common question but the answer will vary between people retiring. For some people the thought of going to work each day becomes overwhelming while for others they have set a retirement date and they are working towards that date. This may not be related to age, such as reaching 65, but could be related to achieving a certain milestone such as 20-30 years with your employer.

For those that have been keen to climb the corporate ladder, being overlooked for more senior roles may trigger the thought of retirement. For some, changes in technology or policies within the organisation may lead to a feeling of 'I am past this' or 'I don't need this any longer'. For others that get involved in social committees such as a golf club, they see a greater sense of fulfilment and being needed than they do at work so the sense of identity shifts from the workplace to the clubhouse. For others there may be a shift from work to grandchildren and community.

These thoughts may result in an almost immediate decision to retire.

While it is good to consult friends and family to get ideas regarding retirement, do not be influenced by being told you are too young or 'why do you want to retire?'. The decision when to retire is yours.

Have you thought about what you may call yourself in retirement? Not everyone likes being called a retiree. Talking with some friends recently, some liked being called retirees, others preferred the term 'self-funded retiree' and some hadn't really thought about it. At some stage in retirement, the question regarding occupation will come up. What occupation will you put on the immigration form when travelling overseas?

Chapter 6

Reinventing yourself

A man is not old until regrets take the place of dreams.
John Barrymore

Are you or your partner one of these people where work is all-consuming to the detriment of all other activities? You may say that is not me but think about what other activities you have outside of work and you may find that it <u>is</u> you.

You spend years learning and preparing for your profession, earning a reputation for your knowledge and expertise as well as the respect of your workmates and then, one day, you are retired.

Unfortunately, our parents' generation didn't provide a real role model for retirement. Previous generations of men had little expectation for retirement, maybe a couple of years to live after working from a very young age. For women, it was possibly harder as they had to give up work when they got married so they never really retired. Their 'retirement' was shaped by their husband's retirement just as their identity was shaped by their husband's occupation.

It has been a long-held belief that men have a tougher time than women adjusting to retirement because, for many, their identity is exclusively tied to their employment and they have few social networks outside of work. Today, women invest just as much time in their careers as men but, even today, women seem to handle retirement better. This is likely due to the fact that women are generally more sociable than men and develop better networks.

Many people don't want to be identified as retired because there is still the image of a retired person sitting at home, doing very little. After years of seeing yourself and being seen by others as a policeman, engineer, nurse, mechanic or whatever your profession was, do you now want to be known as an ex-policeman or ex-professional? You trained and became qualified in your profession so you will always be a nurse, solicitor or mechanic even though you may not practise in that field in retirement.

It is important for your self-esteem (and sometimes for ease of completing government papers such as immigration cards when travelling), to have an identity in retirement. The best time to develop such a new identity is in the lead-up to your retirement rather than waiting for retirement to establish new interests and activities which will contribute to your new identity. In the year or two before you retire, think about yourself without work, structure and the routine that work provides. Start visualising a typical week in retirement after the honeymoon period.

For most people, working for one company for an entire lifetime and then retiring has not been the norm. For many of us, we have wanted to get ahead in our chosen field and often to achieve that promotion has meant changing companies rather than trying to climb the company's corporate ladder. Too often, we were impatient to wait for our next step up the ladder. We have also had to be flexible and prepared to accept a possible change of direction in our career to move forward.

So it is with retirement. The things that you start out doing in your retirement years or even dream about prior to retirement will change over the years and may be radically different from your original dreams. These changes may be brought about by a change in your interests, possibly a change in your marital status, your health or your financial position. So you need to be flexible and also accept that some changes are inevitable.

Initially, you may have a number of projects planned for the period immediately after retirement; specific projects around the house that have been put off until more time is available or more money from a lump sum payment, the extended vacation, cleaning and decluttering the house. Alternatively, you may do little else but play golf or spend time in the garden every day. It is your retirement so you should be able to do what makes you happy.

In retirement, status becomes less relevant as does what you wear. In your career, you may have been a highly respected barrister and wore fashionable suits but in retirement who may care? No longer do you have to wear clothes that are expected of you and your position. No longer do you need status or have people seeking you out for what you may be able to do for them. Some may want to retain such status so they continue working or join a club with the intention of being president or secretary for the status. Most want a simple life, being accepted for who they are as a person and being able to dress as they wish. Have you thought of what your life in retirement may be like?

At parties and other social functions, people may find you far more interesting to talk to about things that you are passionate about than what your employment is or had been. What are you passionate about that may form your new identity?

Below are a few ideas that you could consider for reinventing yourself. It is likely that you may reinvent yourself a number of times during retirement.

Volunteering

Volunteering both before retirement and after retirement has beneficial effects on your adjustment to retirement. Volunteering allows you to try something new, gain experience, develop new skills or utilise existing skills as well as meet new people and give back to the community. It has a number of health benefits such as lowering stress levels, building confidence and giving yourself a sense of meaning and appreciation. Several studies have indicated that volunteers live longer.

According to the 2016 Census, some 3.6 million people had volunteered in 2015. Some areas that people volunteer in are sport, education and training, community and welfare organisations. For charities, volunteering can reduce operating costs like wages for the organisation.

Some of the reasons people volunteer are:

1. to help others,
2. to find a purpose,
3. wanting to make a difference,
4. to give structure to the week,
5. keeping involved,
6. keeping the brain active,
7. to benefit from personal development,
8. to learn more about oneself,
9. to connect with community,
10. learning new skills,
11. using skills in a productive way,
12. exploring new areas of interest,
13. meeting new people of different ages,
14. to escape from negative feelings

Depending on the area chosen, it can be challenging. The challenges can be many such as difficulties in communication, emotional or physical.

Women are more likely than men to volunteer. There are a number of organisations that can put you in touch with organisations seeking volunteers, male and female, including those seeking volunteers to work overseas.

There are hundreds of areas that you can volunteer in so look for one that best suits you. Always check to see if any special skills are required, if any training is provided and whether the hours are flexible enough to allow for family commitments and holiday travel as well.

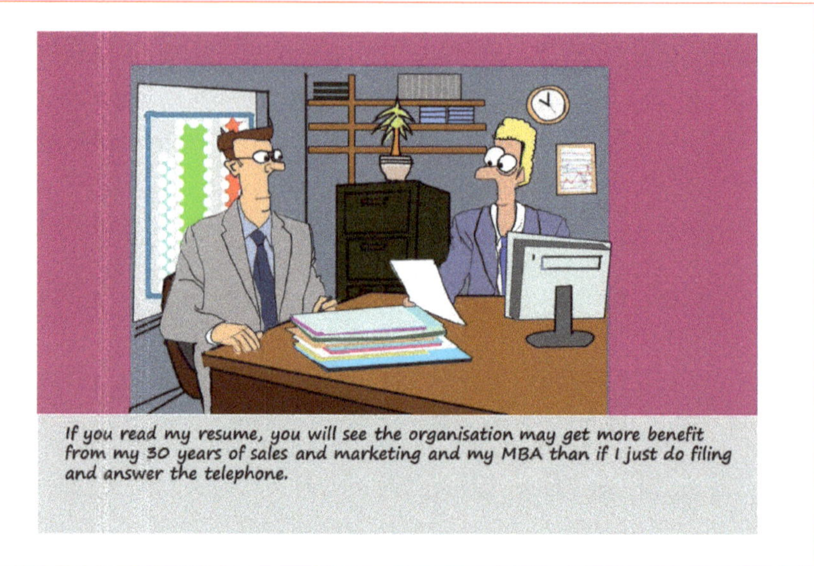

Grandparenting

It is often an overlooked area but one that can lead to conflict within the marriage and among children. A growing number of our adult children are deciding not to have any children or to delay having children until later in life. The latter case means that, unlike our grandparents who may have been in their fifties when grandchildren came along, we are more likely to be in our sixties by the time grandchildren arrive.

Some people thoroughly enjoy their role as a grandparent and their new world appears to revolve around their grandchildren, all other activities taking a back seat; I think that we can all identify with someone like that. This can lead to conflict with their partner if they do not have a shared understanding of the time that will be devoted to looking after grandchildren.

Some people are very happy to reinvent themselves as grandparents and embrace this new identity. They may have a number of grandchildren and a large part of their week is devoted to looking after them. With more than 64 per cent of two-parent families in Australia both working, grandparents may provide full day-care, drop-offs and pickups, or help with after-school care. During school holidays, grandparents provide vacation care and during the school term may transport grandchildren to and from extra-curricular activities as well as attend school events such as concerts, fetes and speech nights. Grandparents are often on call to help with after hours care when parents wish to attend evening functions or events. According to the Australian Bureau of Statistics figures, in 2014 approximately 837,000 children received childcare from their grandparents. In a recent article, it was estimated that grandparents saved their children $2.29 billion a year in childcare costs.

In return, grandparents benefit from building a closer bond with their grandchildren, it helps to connect the family and there are mental and emotional benefits to be gained.

Household duties
While not an area that you would normally associate with a chapter on reinventing yourself, it is relevant.

Spouses or partners in a long-term relationship generally have developed certain household duties that they see as their sole responsibility while there are others that are shared. With retirement, particularly if partners retire at different times, there can be a significant change in these household duties.

As an example, the husband has retired before the wife. This can create tension because of the wife's expectation that their retired partner can now undertake additional duties around the house such as cleaning, washing, cooking and other domestic tasks. Later when the wife retires, she may unconsciously start to undertake some or all of the roles that the husband had previously undertaken. Alternatively, the husband may now decide that since the wife has retired, he no longer needs to do any of the domestic duties. Neither situation is ideal. Both are likely to lead to tension in the household.

It is best to have worked through who will do what household duties before the first partner retires and review it again before the other partner retires to see if there needs to be any adjustments due to new activities being undertaken in retirement.

The second reason why it is important to consider household duties occurs as we get older. It is important that we have some cross skilling of these household duties in case one partner:

1. becomes ill,
2. unable to perform some work due to complaints like arthritis,
3. ends the relationship or
4. passes away.

We all depend to some extent on our partner in certain areas so cross skilling will take some of the burden off each other. We are not suggesting a change of roles; partners can continue doing the duties that they like. It is just a matter of being prepared.

On the last page of this chapter is a draft of the division of household duties that you can work through, adding or deleting tasks as appropriate.

Carer

Some people retire to look after their aged parents or an ill partner or child. It can be both rewarding but emotionally and physically draining so it is important to have a supportive network around you.

Turning skills and hobbies into businesses

Become an author. It is said that there is a book inside everyone so what are you interested in: fiction, non-fiction, children's books, cook books or garden books? Do you want to write a book on your family history? Writing a book and self-publishing a book is relatively easy and inexpensive today.

Start blogging or podcasting if you have a lifestyle, interest or passion that may be of interest to others. There are blogs and podcasts on every conceivable topic now. You never know how large a following you may create in a relatively short period of time.

Teaching or tutoring allows you to use specific skills to develop an online course. There is almost no limit on what you can develop online courses for, whether it is how to knit, sew, assemble flat pack furniture, cooking, gardening or how to fly a plane. As well as the online course, you could become a tutor either in person or online. Have you thought about teaching English to migrants?

Become a consultant using your skills and experience. A consultancy may be possible in certain industries in the lead-up to retirement and in a few years after retirement. Ongoing, it is a matter of keeping your education and skills current.

Have you considered converting a hobby into a small business? Often time and money has kept your hobby a hobby even though people have shown an interest in what you do. Some may want to learn how to do your hobby or they may want to purchase the product. Now, with time and money, can your hobby become a small business? Could you be a photographer, build web sites, make jewellery or use carpentry skills to make furniture and toys?

Gardening can also become a rewarding retirement activity whether it is growing vegetables or flowers. Gardening has some personal benefits in that it can help with your vitamin D intake, benefit your mental health as well as cut down on your grocery bills. Any surplus of produce could be swapped, given away or sold. Your skills may lead you to becoming an expert in your field such as grafting, propagation or composting.

Self-employed

Many of us may have had ambitions of being self-employed but family commitments constrained us from undertaking any such venture. In retirement, your ambitions of being an entrepreneur may become a reality. You have the resources available now that previously you may not have had. There are many options available.

If you have a relatively new car, you could become a self-employed driver for one or more of the ride-share companies like Uber or Didi.

It is relatively inexpensive to establish a business on Amazon for selling a great variety of products. If you believe the information that promoters provide, you buy a cheap product for say $1 per unit and sell it on Amazon for $20 per unit, sometimes with no requirement to hold a large quantity of the product.

Maybe you have had ambitions of starting a coffee shop or secretarial service.

Part time work

One way to prepare for retirement is to reduce the number of hours that you currently work, maybe initially by a day per week and then as retirement gets closer, reducing your working days still further. Depending upon the industry, you may be able to retire, take an extended holiday and then come back to work part time with your current employer.

Other people look to part time work in retirement to supplement their income as well as provide a means to meet people and stay connected. Unfortunately, reality may mean that not everyone that seeks part time work in retirement will be successful.

It is important to remember that any paid work may impact any pension you receive as well as your status as a retiree and access to your superannuation. Understand how much you can earn and the number of hours that you can work.

Identity or status in retirement does not have to be related to money or power or any of those things that status and identity were identified with in employment.

Do you know your purpose in life?

Division of household duties				
Task	Current	Scale of 1 – 5 for like/dislike	Scale of 1 – 5 for competency	Future
Grocery shopping				
Preparing meals				
Setting table				
Washing dishes / stacking dishwasher				
Cleaning kitchen				
Laundry				
Ironing				
Vacuuming				
Washing floors				
Cleaning bathroom / toilets				
Taking rubbish bins out				
Lawn mowing				
Gardening				
Repairs around the house				
Car washing				
Paying bills				
Keeping financial records				
Preparing tax return information				
Buying presents for family and friends				
Buying new clothes				
Knowing how to budget				
Understanding investment portfolio				
System for paying and filing bills				

Key learnings from this chapter

Chapter 7

Health

The secret to living well and longer is: eat half, walk double, laugh triple and love without measure.

- Tibetan Proverb

Age is an issue of mind over matter. If you don't mind, it doesn't matter.

- Mark Twain

Most people will focus on the financial aspects leading up to retirement. This is important but the Australian Government has put in place a safety net in the form of a pension if we do not achieve sufficient to live on in retirement. For your most valuable asset, your health, there is Medicare. Unfortunately, you may have to wait years for surgery and who wants to do that particularly if you are in pain or unable to enjoy any quality of life? There is little point in having a million dollars in a bank account if you are too ill or incapacitated to be able to enjoy what it could provide.

Up to around 50 years of age, most of us, particularly males, have little, if anything, to do with the medical system. We may break a bone or have a serious cut that requires suturing or, most commonly, an infection that needs antibiotics. We fix the current issue but seldom have a complete check-up. On the rare occasion that I have visited a doctor, the doctor complains that they would go broke if they had to rely on patients like me. It has been said that Australians look after their cars better than they do themselves; most Australians neglect to have regular health check-ups.

Like your finances, your health should not be left until retirement. Ideally, you should be looking after your health all through your life but few of us do that. The longevity that we look forward to is also likely to come with some form of disability. The risk of chronic health problems increases, naturally, as you age. Seventy per cent of older people are overweight or obese, 1 in 5 Australians aged 65 and over experience a disability that limits activity, and 87 per cent aged 65 and older have at least one chronic condition. Only 17.2 per cent of older Australians meet the physical activity guidelines. There are things that you can do to reduce or slow the risk. Being active throughout your life is the best way to maintain a healthy well-being and quality of life. An active lifestyle helps prevent and manage chronic conditions, reduces the risk of falls as balance is improved, maintains brain function and memory, helps one stay socially connected and independent.

Around the age of 50, you should make sure that you see your family doctor for an annual check-up. You may find that your doctor may also be preparing for retirement by reducing the hours or days that they attend the practice and particularly if they are in a practice with a number of other doctors. Now may be a time to consider looking for a new doctor, a younger doctor that is likely to be practising as a doctor for many years or at least for your lifetime. Consider whether they have any specific areas of interest or specialities and whether these areas align with the potential care that you may require in the future.

It is a good time to find out what are the important things to get checked and how regularly. It would be helpful if you knew a little of your family health history including any major illnesses that your parents had, what your grandparents died from, and any illnesses that your siblings may have? I went to the State Government Department for Births, Deaths and Marriages and obtained death certificates for my parents, grandparents and great-grandparent so that I had some idea of what they died from. It is worth discussing this information with your doctor because sometimes there may be multiple diseases put down as a cause of death but, in reality, they would not have caused the death. One of the causes of my grandfather's death listed was glaucoma. Yes, he had suffered from glaucoma for a number of years but it did not result in his death. I was upset when I read the causes of death for my great-grandfather, one of which was malnutrition. I knew very well that my grandparents, with whom he lived, would not have allowed this to occur. Later I found out that, back then, it was common for this to occur in hospitals for older people with terminal illnesses or 'old age'.

As you age, you may start to show signs of some chronic conditions like high blood pressure, high cholesterol or high sugar levels as well as arthritis or digestive problems. So you move from the quick fix to managing the problems over the next couple of decades. It is also possibly the period in which some serious health issues in terms of strokes, heart attacks and cancers may present. You need to consider how you wish to deal with these illnesses because we know that these conditions can present at any age. In the past, you might have thought that it would happen to someone else and so dismiss the possibility. Unfortunately, as we age, the probability is likely to increase.

This is true of older people being more susceptible to cancer and scientists have yet to understand why. It could be that the body is less able to repair cells or a longer exposure to cancer-causing agents. A healthy lifestyle appears to lower the possibility of cancers. Losing weight, regular exercise and a good diet are part of a healthy lifestyle.

There have been countless advertising campaigns over our lifetime to stop smoking. If you are still smoking, now is the time to stop for good. Stopping smoking is the single best thing that can be done to improve your health and potential longevity. There is a link between smoking and dementia, cataracts, heart stroke and lung disease but, one year after quitting, chances of smoke-related diseases drop by almost 50 percent.

A person may not realise it but our body changes the way it can handle alcohol. Drinking in moderation is now more important than previously. The recommended alcohol limit is one drink per day for females and two drinks per day for males.

We are often told that exercise and diet are important for good health, and it certainly is, but we must also look after our mind...

Mind

While at work, there are problems to solve and other activities to stimulate our mind. In retirement, there may not be such stimulation. It is important that you look to pursue activities that will exercise your brain and there is no better time to start than now.

It is normal to have some memory loss as you age as the brain appears to store information in a slightly different way. What is not normal is not being able to follow simple directions or forgetting the way home. This could be a sign of a medical condition such as dementia or Alzheimer's disease.

Our brain is like a muscle and the more that it is exercised, the better condition it will retain. Challenging the mind can improve brain function and our overall health. So what can you do to challenge your mind?

You may decide to learn a new language, particularly if you plan to travel or maybe undertake a house swap. You may decide to learn a musical instrument or even undertake a new hobby. For example, a friend of mine has learnt to construct a guitar and is now learning to play this guitar.

Playing cards, (Bridge is a good example) or doing a crossword, puzzles, jigsaws, word searches or Sudoku are all good for challenging the brain. Daily newspapers have some of these crosswords, word searches and Sudoku games, and there are others available in book format as well as online. There is also a great variety of board games such as chess, checkers and mahjong. You will also find online various quizzes covering your knowledge of such areas as history, geography, sport, science, music and general knowledge. Whether you are good or bad to start, patience and persistence will help.

Mental health is often overlooked but it is more important as we age. Depression and anxiety are common as people age and can be a result of chronic disease, chronic pain, social isolation, multiple personal losses, lifestyle changes and reduced independence.

Staying in touch with friends and family is good as loneliness can cause depression. Why not join a book club, perhaps write a book or simply go for a walk with a friend regularly?

Both our mental and physical health can be severely affected when suffering from stress, anxiety or depression. Mental illness includes anxiety, depression, schizophrenia, bipolar affective disorder and personality disorders. Mental illness can have an impact on a person's cognitive, behavioural and social functioning resulting in social isolation. Too often, the symptoms can be dismissed but it is important to talk to people about what is causing your stress and anxiety to avoid loneliness. Sadly 1 in 5 Australians will experience a mental illness. As a nation, we have a poor understanding and acceptance of mental illness to the extent that it often goes undiagnosed, poorly treated or even untreated.

There is growing evidence suggesting exercise is an effective treatment method for people suffering from acute and chronic mental illness. Some studies have suggested exercise is just as effective as pharmacological intervention in alleviating depression symptoms but this needs to be discussed with your doctor before undertaking any action. Aerobic exercise and weight-lifting are good but so is swimming, riding a bike, bushwalking and yoga.

Consideration can also be given to relaxation music, meditation, tai chi or even owning a pet? Pets are shown to be therapeutic as they are great companions and, if the pet is a dog, it provides a good reason to go for a walk.

Next we will look at what makes a healthy body because a healthy body makes a huge difference to mental attitude and cognitive ability.

Body

One does not have to be a gym junkie or pound the pavement each day to enjoy good health and remain fit. But, more than ever, good health is important. Lifestyle, environment and genetics are three of the main factors affecting mortality statistics. Lifestyle represents more than 50 per cent and it is one factor that we can influence. In the chapter on finances, we looked at ways of reducing costs. An investment in a healthy lifestyle now will mean lower medical costs and a longer period of independent living in the future. Numerous research papers have shown that people who live longer, are sick less often, and enjoy happier lives, all have a regime of regular exercise.

One in five Australians will suffer chronic pain and this number increases to 1 in 3 after the age of 65. About 16 per cent of the Australian population have back problems and between 70–90 per cent of people will suffer from lower back pain at some point in their life. One in three Australian men over the age of 50 is on pain medication.

While we are working, most of us are getting some form of exercise. It may not necessarily be the recommended 10,000 steps per day but there is a considerable number achieved by doing simple things like walking to and from public transport on the way to work, walking to the conference room for meetings, to the coffee shop for a coffee, maybe a walk at lunch time to shop for clothes and then the return trip home. These steps do tend to mount up but what will happen in retirement?

Now is the time to start thinking about how active you may be in retirement and starting a routine for exercise. We are not necessarily promoting a visit to the gym five days per week (although that would be fantastic) but, as a minimum, try just walking around the streets of your neighbourhood for about 20–30 minutes. Walking, particularly brisk walking, is a most effective exercise. It can be a gentle pace to start but if there are some areas that are a little hilly, try to include some parts of this in your exercise. If it is a flat area, is there some part that you might be able to jog or walk briskly for a small distance to get your heart rate up and to add some variety? Try not to let bad weather deter exercise. If it is raining, why not go to the local shopping centre like a Westfields and walk around the shopping centre for 30 minutes? (Walking with an umbrella is another option but this is not as effective since you will be unable to swing both arms). Studies have shown that walking three times a week for about 30 minutes each time can increase life expectancy, help with better sleep and reduce rates of cancer, diabetes and depression.

Anyone for tennis, golf, swimming or bowls? Consider being a coach for your children's or grandchildren's little athletics, cricket, football or hockey teams. Also, have you considered pilates, yoga classes or dancing?

It may take a little time for it to become a matter of routine, so start now. Set short term realistic goals for exercising each week. Write your exercise plan down and try to exercise at a specific time each day, one that fits in with your lifestyle. This helps to form a habit. A person that I go to gym with exercises 5 days a week at 7 am so the exercise is done and the rest of the day is free. The best time to exercise is when you have the most energy and motivation. Even just getting up from a chair and moving around for 2 minutes every 30 minutes is worthwhile exercise.

If you are away on a business trip, try to fit in a 30-minute walk around the city streets or visit the gym if the hotel has one.

Gyms are good providing that there is a qualified person to develop a program suitable for your needs. Prior to starting at a gym, have an assessment undertaken and then an individual program developed for you that meets your exercise goals. You need to monitor your muscle and joint soreness after each session and, while some soreness is to be expected, notify your gym instructor if you feel it is excessive. It is important to establish the proper training loads and progressively increase them as your muscle strength improves. Your gym instructor should show you how to use the equipment correctly and then regularly check on you to make sure that you are doing your exercises correctly. Gyms make their money out of gym memberships so, generally, they are not concerned whether you attend or not. Find a partner to go to the gym with and then you can hold each other accountable.

People who decide to do exercise generally focus on the cardiovascular to ward off potential heart issues but, as you age, you need to look also at flexibility and balance plus resistance training. Cardio exercise benefits the heart by decreasing fat, lowers blood pressure and gains muscle mass and strength. Along with other forms of exercise it helps reduce anxiety and depression. For maximum benefit, any exercise should be combined with an appropriate diet as your energy breakdown is increased by more physical exercise.

As you age, you will lose flexibility and elasticity and your body mass will decrease. Inflexibility is a significant contributor to physical deterioration so it is important to include some flexibility exercises in your overall fitness program. Some people will, and you should, include some simple stretching exercises both before and after aerobic and resistance exercises but there should also be a separate component designed to improve your flexibility.

Another part of any fitness program should involve strength and resistance training to help build muscle mass and increase metabolism. Through the use of weights, resistance machines, press-ups etc, your goal should be to tone your body not to bulk up excessively. Weights do not need to be heavy initially as you are likely to build up to heavier weights. The key is small but consistent increases in the amount of weight lifted and repetition of each exercise. Exercise reduces your risk of falling by building muscle strength and helps control body weight and blood pressure.

Regular, light weightlifting will not only increase your physical strength and resilience but also your attitudinal and internal strength. Other benefits of strength and resistance training include prevention of muscle loss associated with aging, increased lean muscle mass, increased bone density and joint health, and a reduced risk of some chronic diseases. It will also improve sleep and mental health. Studies have shown that strength and resistance training has the potential to reduce the risk of dementia, Alzheimer's and Parkinson's disease.

Other simple exercises that involve balance are also worth doing. For example, standing on one leg, use the other leg to move to points to the north, east, south and west.

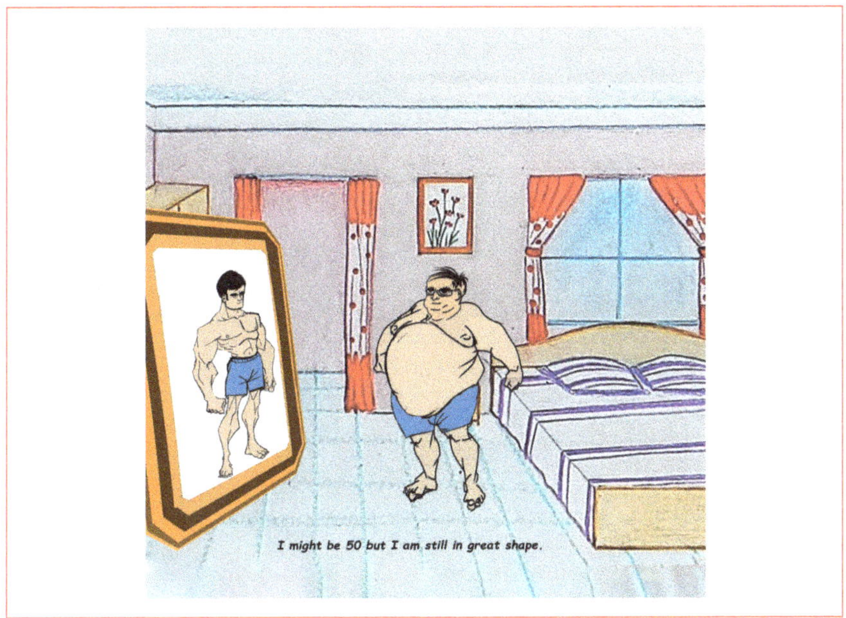

At home, we are generally less active now than we were 40 or 50 years ago. Today, we sit in our armchairs and change the channel on our television with a remote control compared with having to get out of the chair to change the channel by rotating a dial. Even your use of a telephone has changed how you move. Fifty years ago, there were no mobile phones so it was either walking down the hallway to the phone on the wall or, if the house had no phone, walking down the street to the public phone box.

If you wanted groceries, you had to walk to the corner store. Today, you use your car to drive to the supermarket or, more recently, order online and then the supermarket delivers to the house. Not much effort is required there – our modern lifestyle is causing us harm.

Sleep patterns often change as you get older; you sleep earlier and wake earlier. People often accept that you need less sleep as you age but the reality is that you need between seven and nine hours of sleep each night. Some health conditions that have been linked to not getting sufficient sleep include memory problems, depression and night-time falls. Regardless of age, we all need good sleep but the length of sleep may vary. If you are having trouble sleeping, you are more tired than may be expected, or you wake up feeling tired, then talk to your doctor.

As you age, your metabolism slows; you burn fewer calories than when you were younger for the same amount of activity. You may have less energy and you put on weight. Once you have put on the weight, it is difficult to lose it. What is the healthy weight range for your height? Is the ratio of waist-to-hip measurement acceptable or has it changed? If your waist size has increased compared to your hip then there could be an increased risk of health problems like diabetes. Obesity can increase the chances of heart disease, stroke, diabetes, high blood pressure, arthritis and some thirteen different types of cancer including breast, colon and pancreatic cancers.

Your immune system isn't as strong when you get older. Seniors represent the majority of people who die or are hospitalised from serious flu-related complications like pneumonia, heart/lung disease and sepsis, which is a bacterial infection in the blood. It is for these reasons that a yearly vaccination is recommended.

For 40-year old males, there is a 1 in 2 risk of developing coronary heart disease. Every year, some 26,000 Australians suffer heart attacks, 23,000 develop malignant cancers and 18,000 suffer strokes. Stroke is the leading cause of long-term disability in adults.

The average life expectancy for an Australian is currently 82 but, for some, the last ten years or so can be completely dysfunctional.

A fear of falling is unfortunately something that increases with age and we often hear about seniors falling and breaking bones. Osteoporosis, a disease causing extremely low bone density, affects 1 in 3 women over the age of 50. (*The Burden of Brittle Bones: Epidemiology, Costs and Burden of Osteoporosis in Australia 2007*). Over 2.2 million Australians (men and women) over the age of 50 are affected by osteoporosis. There are no symptoms before the first fracture so it is important to have a scan to determine a baseline bone density. A bone mineral density scan gives a 'T' score which represents the density of the bone. Using this T score, the bone health is classified into osteoporosis, osteopenia or normal. The results may indicate whether dietary or other treatment options should be considered. Recent research has indicated that exercise, particularly resistance training, can increase bone density.

Osteoarthritis, not to be confused with osteoporosis, occurs when the cartilage between the joints breaks down. It normally starts after 40 years of age and most people are likely to suffer from it in a normal life span. Osteoarthritis can cause pain and stiffness in knees, hips, neck and hands. There is a correlation between injuries to joints as we grew up, genes inherited from parents, body weight and diet.

As you age, you see the outward signs, more wrinkles, more grey hair (if you have any hair at all), and your body shape changes with a tendency to replace lean body mass (muscle) with fat, particularly around the stomach. The natural aging process also leads to distinct loss of muscle mass and strength with about a 15 per cent loss per decade over the age of 50. This is a result of many factors such as insufficient nutrient intake, muscle atrophy, decreased physical activity, and loss of anabolic factors such as growth hormones, androgens and estrogens. Chronic conditions such as heart disease and rheumatoid arthritis also play a part.

Your body is also aging on the inside and developing health issues.

Some areas that you need to check include:

- Blood pressure, cholesterol and triglycerides levels
- Glucose levels, particularly if there is a family history of diabetes
- Weight and Body Mass Index (BMI) which can lead to a higher incidence of high blood pressure, cholesterol and glucose.
- Prostate check (males)
- Skin (for sun cancers, moles)
- Thyroid levels
- Osteoporosis
- Colorectal cancer
- Vision and hearing
- Screening for breast, colon and cervical cancers (females)
- A review of your family history looking for any hereditary health issues.

Medical science has come a long way in the last few decades but it is better to remain healthy and avoid medical intervention. Prevention is important as it leads to a better quality of life and saves you (and the economy) thousands and thousands of dollars in medical procedures, hospital beds, recuperation time and stress for all concerned.

Before leaving this section, consider booking yourself and your partner in to undertake a first aid course. It may come in handy attending to minor cuts and abrasions with grandchildren but, more importantly, your first aid knowledge may save someone's life – maybe your partner's.

Diet

Relax – we are not going to talk about starting a strict diet; there are many books in the bookstores or online to choose from. Just over 70 per cent of all deaths are attributable to heart disease, cancer and diabetes and diet can have a major impact on these. You do need to recognise that, as you grow older, your body needs different foods and that you can no longer eat the same food, or quantity of food, that you once did.

It is important to monitor not only your weight but also your BMI to keep them within acceptable limits for your age and height.

You have heard the advertising campaigns that governments have run in terms of how many servings of fresh fruit and vegetables you should have per day. How many of us have actually applied this to the way we eat? A national health survey found that only 8 per cent of adults were eating the 5 servings of vegetables per day and only 48 per cent were eating the 2 servings of fruit per day. Perhaps in compensation, about 25 per cent of Australians use a vitamin or mineral supplement.

In addition, you should reduce your intake of red meat and processed foods and increase the fish, particularly oily fish, in your diet. Eating lots of fruit and vegetables and foods high in calcium helps keep your bones stronger.

Drinking water is good as it not only keeps the body hydrated but makes you go to the toilet more often and lessens the likelihood of kidney stones.

It is worth keeping a record of what you eat and drink for a fortnight and then consult a dietician to see if there are any changes that need to be made to your diet.

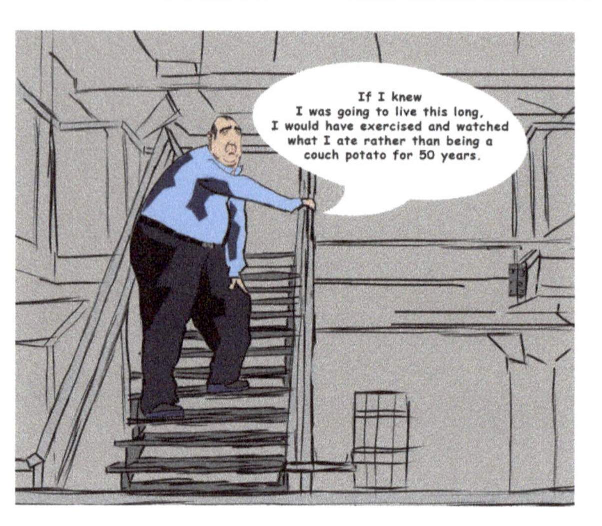

Health supplements

Australian chemists and supermarkets have aisles packed with vitamins, minerals and other supplements. There is a market for them but is the Australian public being hoodwinked? The Australian pharmaceutical industry is large but it is the supplements industry that has some people concerned. An investigation by the ABC Four Corners program in 2017 reported that over 60 per cent of all Australians use some type of supplement and the Australian complementary medicine industry is reported to have revenue of $4.7 billion in 2016, a $1.2 billion increase since 2014. The investigation was into the effectiveness and safety of supplements. Complementary medicines are not tested and regulated to the same level as prescription drugs and they can interact with other prescribed medicines in unforeseen ways.

There are certain groups for whom complementary medicines may be beneficial. These include people with a disease affecting the absorption of nutrients such as coeliac disease, those with a specific nutrient deficiency and those who cannot eat enough food to meet their nutrient requirements. For those with a specific nutrient deficiency such as vitamin D, iron or vitamin

B12, supplements are useful to bring nutrient levels up to normal but then diet should be sufficient to maintain levels. As well as the elderly, some say that vegetarians and vegans may not eat enough of a balanced diet to meet their nutrient requirements and therefore need to take vitamin and mineral supplements.

So what are some of the common types of supplements?

Calcium and vitamin D are taken to strengthen bones and prevent osteoporosis but, for average Australians, recent studies indicate they get sufficient calcium from milk and vitamin D from exposure to sunlight. People with no dairy intake and people with little exposure to sunlight, (like the elderly confined to bed in a nursing home) would benefit. However, if you have one glass of milk per day and spend some time in the sun, it is unlikely that you will need this supplement.

Fish oil capsules containing omega 3 essential fatty acids and are used to prevent heart disease, arthritis and immune system disorder. Some research has shown that fish oil supplements reduce triglycerides but not the risk of heart attack, or stroke. In 2015, the Heart Foundation updated its position statement by saying there was insufficient evidence to support the use of fish oil supplements in preventing heart attacks and that there also seemed little difference between liquid and capsule fish oil – but it depended upon the quality of the product. The Heart Foundation recommends 2-3 serves of oily fish per week. Salmon, sardines, mackerel, tuna, trout and mullet are examples of oily fish.

Vitamin C acts as an antioxidant, helps grow and repair tissue within the body and prevents scurvy. Vitamin C is found in kale, citrus fruits, berries and peas. The main evidence seems to indicate that using a vitamin C supplement reduces the duration of a cold.

Glucosamine is derived from crab, lobster or shrimp shells and is used as a treatment for osteoarthritis. There have been mixed studies and a combination of glucosamine sulfate and chondroitin sulfate may improve pain and reduce the narrowing of joint space.

There have been many calls for herbal remedies to be independently tested as some remedies have been found to contain natural toxins, heavy metals or pesticides. Since 2011, at least six organ transplants that have been required in Australia have been linked to herbal supplements. One, in 2016, when a West Australian lost his liver, was most likely the result of taking a protein powder containing a green tea extract.

The natural variations of herbal supplements mean it is difficult to ensure consistency.

Cranberry, in the form of juice, tablets and capsules, has been used to treat and prevent urinary tract infections. However, studies do not support this use particularly for capsules or tablets. The drinking of juice could help treat a urinary tract infection by flushing out the system but it is claimed drinking lots of water could achieve the same result.

Echinacea is used to treat colds and respiratory tract infections but the limited research has shown only a small benefit. However, there are concerns that it causes gastrointestinal problems, allergic reactions and increased asthma.

St John's wort is used to treat depression and there is evidence to support the efficacy of the plant for mild to moderate depression but not major depression. It does, however, interact with many common drugs so its use should be discussed with your doctor prior to using it. Some of the known interactions with common medications include a reduced effect of blood thinning drugs (for example Warfarin), increased risk of side effects if used with antidepressants, increased risk of side effects if used with Triptan migraine medicines and lessening the effect of epilepsy medications.

Vitamin and mineral supplements can never be a substitute for a healthy and varied diet as science cannot replicate exactly what is contained in the food we eat – particularly the phytochemicals from plants. Vitamins and supplements also cannot provide the fibre contained in food.

Complementary and alternative medicines

There has been an expanding following of alternative medicine for the last few decades. The age groups that most use complementary medicines are the 50–59, followed by 60–69 and then 40–49.

Some people do not like the idea of being on prescribed drugs for the rest of their lives. They look for 'natural' alternatives whether in the form of natural medicines or other forms of therapies. Unfortunately, too often they start the 'natural alternatives' without advising their doctor. As you have read in the health supplements section, some of these supplements can have side effects or reduce the benefits of other medicines being taken.

This is where you need to develop a philosophy as to what type of medical treatment you want in the future. You need to seek information from various sources, not just friends or people with a (perhaps uninformed) bias.

The types of complementary medicine that are current include chiropractic, acupressure, acupuncture, energy therapies like Reiki and hypnosis, movement practices like yoga and tai chi, spiritual practices like prayer or meditation, therapeutic massage and traditional Chinese or Ayurvedic medicine.

As with any medical intervention, there has to be understanding and common sense applied and, if in doubt, obtain a second opinion.

There are an increasing number of general practitioners trained in conventional western medicine that are also trained in, or embrace, some alternative medicines. They are therefore able to offer their patients the best of both approaches.

It is your body so you need to discuss with your doctor the medication and treatment and, if considering alternative methods, how these may interact with any prescribed medication and the possible side effects of ceasing certain medications.

Chapter 8

Where will you live?

*The house of everyone is to him his castle and fortress. **Sir Edward Coke 1604** now simplified to A man's home is his castle.*

Retirement may mean a change in where we live. It may be a chance to downsize to a smaller home or to move to the country or seaside for that long-awaited tree change or sea change. For others, it may mean a move into an Over 55s or a retirement village. In this chapter we will look at various options, some of which you may or may not have considered.

During your working life, your place of abode has been dictated primarily by the location of your workplace or a particular school for your children. With retirement, those particular constraints have been removed. New constraints may appear such as a desire to be close to grandchildren or, if parents are still alive, a need to visit and assist them. There is also an expectation with some people that it is a chance to downsize to a smaller house. Downsizing, within the same area, is seldom likely to be financially beneficial.

Rather than wait for retirement and a major relocation, now is the time to be thinking about where you may want to live. You may consider visiting a number of different locations at different times of the year to see what the climate is like and to start developing some connections with the area. You need to psyche yourself up before making such major changes. Despite what you sometimes read in newspapers or see on television, it is only a small percentage of people that opt for a sea change or a tree change.

If you have any thoughts at all of possibly relocating or downsizing then there are a number of things that you need to consider now rather than waiting for retirement.

There is no right or wrong answer and, if you talk to your partner, he/she may also have a very different idea of where to live. Choosing where to live is a very important decision and not one to be taken lightly. A wrong decision could prove extremely costly. The two most costly mistakes are moving from the city to regional or coastal areas and moving too many times. People may move from the city to a regional or coastal area in order to access and use the equity gained towards their retirement. If they decide to move back to the city, property prices in the city may have moved upwards. There are also the various costs associated with buying and selling a property. Moving back to the city then costs more than you originally gained from moving. This is sometimes compounded by the second mistake; that of moving too many times. Sometimes retirees move interstate to a location only to find that they miss their friends and family. Some move multiple times and each of these moves seriously depletes their equity or cashflow. Each move results in furniture relocation costs, buying and selling costs such as agent and legal fees and stamp duty to name a few. Always listen to your head rather than your heart.

It has also been found that relocating after retirement is psychologically much more challenging than retiring and remaining in your home or relocating prior to retirement. Be mindful that there is never an absolutely perfect place that meets every person's requirements.

Personal characteristics
People who relocate are often people with more adventurous personalities, less risk-averse and with a positive attitude towards the future. If people have moved house a few times during their working life, they tend to understand the positive and negative impacts of relocating and therefore have less doubts about moving.

Often, they also have a clear vision of their retirement lifestyle, of living in a different location and the activities they are likely to pursue; for example golf, bowls, fishing or simply reading and gardening.

People that have not become part of the community in which they have lived are more likely to relocate as they have no emotional ties to keep them in that town. People become part of the community by being actively involved and by joining various clubs, being on the school's P&C or being part of the local church. Other people may want to relocate because they feel that the neighbourhood as they remember it has lost its character, traffic has become a problem or too many apartments are being built.

The health of the retiree also has an impact on the decision to relocate. Those with good health may decide that this is the time for them to enjoy life, perhaps even to consider an overseas relocation. Those whose health is not good may decide that it is time to move closer to family, to medical facilities or even look at retirement villages before further health problems or their physical condition deteriorates.

Family home

The family home that your children grew up in may not be the most appropriate home in retirement. You need to spend some time evaluating, unemotionally, how suitable the family home is going to be for you in retirement. It may be suitable at present but what if you had a major illness or reduced mobility? How long will it be liveable? Some long-term planning now could save you a lot of frustration, money and heartache in the future.

How easy would it be to convert your home to address various problems? If the house has stairs, can a lift be installed or a ramp to provide access? Is there an area downstairs that you could convert into a bedroom? You may like gardening but is it manageable or will you need to employ someone to mow the lawn and weed the garden beds? Do you have sufficient funds in retirement to do this? How safe is your home? Good security is important as people get older.

Your house may possibly be too large now for what you require. Is the house going to require a lot of ongoing maintenance?

Do you see this house as an interim step before moving, when you need to, into a retirement village or an aged care facility? You need to look at your existing house with fresh eyes and evaluate it from a different perspective to make conscious decisions.

You also need to consider other factors apart from the physical aspect of the house. How walkable is your suburb? Do you have friends or family close by that may be able to assist in an emergency or can you call on your neighbours? If you are unable to drive a car, how close are the shops and public transport? How well will your existing home serve you in the future as you get older?

It is difficult for most people that may have lived in the family home for 10-20 years to look rationally at the long-term suitability of the family home for retirement. There are accumulations of a lifetime of memories associated with the children growing up in that house. Some people rationalise the need to keep the home as it will be nice when the grandchildren stay over but is that likely?

The home is also the focal point around which people organise their everyday lives and experiences.

When planning your retirement, and particularly where you will live, you need to take a long-term view of at least 10-20 years. Is how you have used your house in the past likely to change in the future? For some people who are handy with tools but have been time-poor, the house is now seen as a never-ending list of maintenance items that they can personally undertake. How old are the floor coverings, the kitchen and appliances? Carrying out renovations or undertaking overdue maintenance a couple of years prior to retirement may be worth considering.

For others, it becomes a project for long-contemplated renovations to be undertaken.

The freedom of retirement may also allow more time for entertaining friends. You may have guests from intrastate, interstate or overseas staying overnight or for a few days. For those keen to travel regularly for extended periods, the house may become a base to return to, to catch up with friends and family, or plan another trip before heading off on the next adventure. The house can also be a museum or art gallery for mementos gathered over the years and on recent trips. Alternatively, those who do not appreciate these mementos may see the house as a place of hoarding for pack rats.

If planning to start or continue in a business after retiring, the house may be an office if undertaking some consultancy type work or even a warehouse if an online business is undertaken.

For others, their home becomes a retreat, an escape from the world. They may have established nice gardens, a good library or a great collection of music and they are happy to interact with the world only when they choose to.

The way you use your home can be a combination of any of these.

You do need to be realistic and consider the long-term suitability of the home.

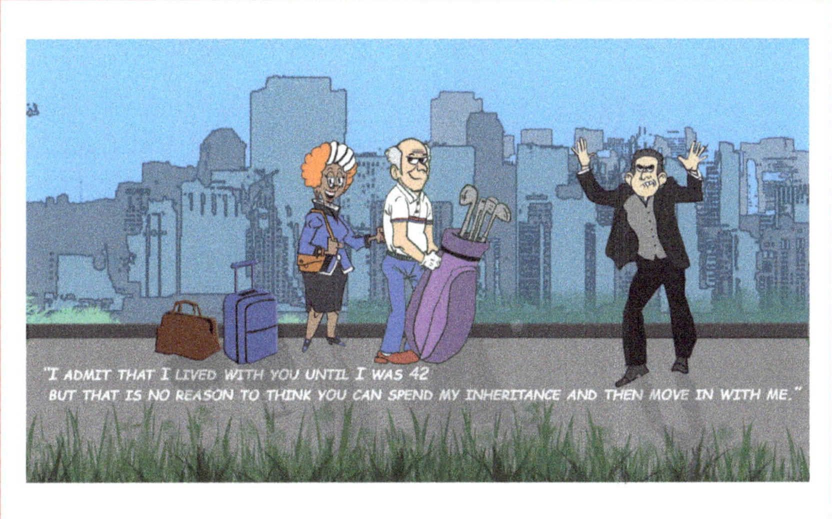

Many retirees are asset rich but income poor with a large portion of their wealth tied up in their home so you need to look at the various options available.

Have you considered building an auxiliary dwelling, commonly called a granny flat, in your backyard? You may decide to live in the granny flat and rent the house out, or vice versa? Can the existing house be modified to create a dual occupancy arrangement? What does your council allow? Is it financially feasible?

Do you wish to have a sea change or a tree change? It may make financial sense to sell the family home and buy in your chosen area. However, what happens if the sea change or tree change has not gone as planned or there are family or health issues and you wish to move back to the city? You are likely to be at a financial disadvantage in finding another house that is unaffordable, particularly in the area where you had previously lived. Why not try renting a house in the sea change or tree change area for six months and see whether this lifestyle lives up to expectations? Talk to an accountant about the six-year rule.

Always allow funds to renovate a property that you buy. Unless it is relatively new, the property is likely to require a new kitchen, appliances, bathroom or painting to be carried out.

If you plan to downsize within a city, it is generally very difficult to find a smaller house in an area with all the facilities and networks that you would like without being financially disadvantaged. The costs associated with selling and buying a house or apartment in Australia makes it a costly exercise. In many cases, downsizing does not become a financially viable option. Real estate agents have promoted the idea of downsizing over many years but the huge numbers expected to downsize are yet to materialise. If planning to relocate, leave yourself sufficient time to declutter. This is not an easy exercise, particularly for a married couple, as there is likely to be differences of opinion as to what should go and what should be kept. You may try to give some items to your children but they or their partners may not want your precious keepsakes. They have little sentimental value to others so consider giving items to an op shop.

You could sell the family home and rent. The Australian Government has recognised this as an option for some people and allows $300,000 to be put into superannuation, providing some conditions are met. You will need to consider the ongoing rental liabilities and make sure that you will have sufficient funds in the future to meet the rent. A drawback here is that you lose some security. You may live in a rental for a long period and, if the landlord sells, you may have to find a new home often at a higher rent. You may consider selling the house to your children who allow you to continue to live there. This may free up cash and allow you to remain in familiar surroundings. Will selling your house have any effect on your pension entitlements? Most contented retirees move no more than 200 kilometres or a two-hour drive from where they had lived.

For a couple of decades, developers of retirement villages, the real estate industry and others with a vested interest, have spoken about the Baby Boomers downsizing. There has been a fear of all the Baby Boomers suddenly selling their large homes, creating a glut and forcing the prices down. Boomers, however, are not following any traditional retirement path. A relatively recent event is the idea of multi-generational housing in Australia. It has been around for centuries overseas but is now becoming more popular in Australia as the price of houses, particularly in the major cities, makes housing less affordable for younger people. New houses are being built with the intention of the house accommodating the grandparents, parents and children. Existing houses, in sought-after suburbs, are being renovated to accommodate multi-generational families. Some large houses are being converted into boarding houses.

If you are a homeowner who may become asset rich but cash poor in retirement, a home loan known as a 'reverse mortgage' may allow you to release the equity in your home. Anyone thinking of a reverse mortgage should discuss the implications with their family. It is such an important topic and one that can cause a lot of concern among family members at a later date. It will affect the value of any future inheritance.

Do you know retirees who have moved to another area or downsized their house? Ask them about their experience.

Holiday house

For many people, owning a holiday house at the beach, in the country or on the snowfields has been a dream. You only have to look at the number of people who look in the windows of real estate agencies while on holidays to see that it is an ambition for many.

The reality is that for many who buy a holiday house, their dreams of getting away on weekends or holiday time does not meet reality. We all live busy lives so it is difficult generally to get away for those weekends. If you decide to let the property out to help meet the costs associated with mortgage, rates and insurance, then you are unable to use the property in peak times when the majority of the income for the property is earned.

Often, the holiday property is put back on the market by a disillusioned owner within a few short years.

But, as retirees, constraints of work are gone so you may now be able to gain those benefits of a holiday house that have possibly eluded you in the past. Would it not be nice to have a place that your children and grandchildren could come to?

Do you move to your favourite holiday destination or do you keep it as your special holiday destination and choose to live in another area?

Explore the possibilities before making any decisions. Visit the destination at different times of the year and in both peak and off-peak seasons.

Overseas destinations

Australians, like our Kiwi neighbours, are great travellers. It is not surprising then that another option becoming popular with retirees is living permanently overseas. As people travel, they find places that they fall in love with such as Bali, Thailand, Cambodia or the Pacific Islands. Also, many Australians return to the home of their birth or ancestry such as New Zealand, Italy, Greece or Spain. Australians are also relocating to some less likely areas including Malaysia, Mexico, Ecuador and Panama.

Some countries like Spain and Portugal entice overseas property buyers with offers of residency permits when they purchase property over a certain value.

The number of Australians over 55 permanently relocating overseas has increased from 7,910 in 2005 to 11,660 in 2016 according to ABS data. For some, there is a benefit in moving to another country as the cost of living and the cost of housing is cheaper. Any thought of relocating overseas will, however, require a lot of consideration and planning.

When thinking of overseas locations as a retirement destination, there are a number of factors that need to be considered. The potential retiree would need to consider primarily the distance from Australia, and family and friends. Do not assume that family and friends will come to visit. They may in the first year or two and then, after that, you may need to undertake the travel. In a family crisis or a death in Australia, how easy will it be to find flights back to Australia and how expensive are those flights?

Notwithstanding the medical tourism that countries like Thailand are becoming known for, is there access to good medical facilities? It may not be important initially but it is something that needs to be considered long-term even if you take great care of your body.

Generally, most countries are politically stable but your individual safety could be of concern while at home or out in the community.

Recently, there was another example of a 54-year-old farmer in South Africa who was stabbed to death in her own home.

Is there any large expat community that you can join, and is English widely spoken, or will you have to learn a language other than English? Is the place popular with retirees? If it is, then it may have the facilities attractive to retirees.

What is the exchange rate like between the Australian dollar and the currency of the country you are considering and is that currency stable? This also needs to be considered if you were to sell and move back to Australia.

If you qualify for an Australian pension, does the country have an agreement with the Australian Government to offer a pension?

Australia is a country without any death duties but that is not the case for other countries. If you have assets in the country that you are thinking of retiring to, does it have death duties and if so what are the death duties applied to? Is it just the assets held in that country, or is it on your entire assets worldwide? Do you understand the taxation system in the country and any reciprocal arrangements with Australia?

Most countries have a capital gains tax but they may also have local taxes that do not exist in Australia; for example property taxes, value added tax applied to any improvements made, wealth tax for property over a certain value, and inheritance taxes.

Before buying overseas, it is prudent to speak with a solicitor based in that country who understands inheritance tax. Is a new will required to be prepared in that country in case you die in that country and your Australian will is not recognised?

Does the country have fast and reliable internet so that you can keep in touch with family and friends by email and Skype as well as undertake internet banking?

Does the country and area have other facilities that you may want like libraries and gyms?

Moving overseas, particularly if you have sold all your property in Australia, can lead to buying a poverty package. This can also happen by buying in other parts of Australia if you are relocating from a capital city but the magnitude of the poverty may be greatly increased if you sell up in Australia, move overseas then have to move back in a few years and buy a house. The price of houses may have increased and you no longer can afford to live in the area that you would like to.

Retirement villages

Firstly, we should differentiate between a retirement village and aged care or rest home. Retirement villages are for independent living while aged care is for people who are no longer able to live independently.

People can move into a retirement village generally from age 55 and some people choose to do so to enjoy the social and physical activities available.

Retirement villages are to be found in many different locations; at the beach, in cities and rural towns. The accommodation style ranges from single or double storey townhouses with small gardens to high-rise apartments and from a small complex of maybe 30 units to large complexes of a few hundred. The facilities that these retirement villages offer vary considerably with libraries, coffee shops, hairdressers, doctors' rooms, swimming pool, bowls and tennis courts – but they generally come at a price.

It may be worth considering a retirement village that has aged care facilities attached so that you are not changing location completely as your care requirements change.

Aged care

The *Australian Financial Review,* 4-5 August 2018, stated that there is a general resistance to moving into an aged care home unless all other options have been tried or assessed.

In the late 1950's and early 1960's, my aunty Anne operated an aged care home in Perth and later in Sydney. This was at a time when most nursing homes or aged care homes were small facilities (approximately 30 beds) operated as family businesses or by not-for-profit organisations. Over time, large companies have taken over the market just as they have done in the funeral industry.

Interestingly, this period of the 1950s and 1960s was the time when large institutions housed orphaned children and people with mental illness or disabilities. Smaller community based services are now the norm following the deinstitutionalisation of these large institutions. Will the current or potentially other Royal Commissions into aged care ultimately result in a deinstitutionalisation of aged care?

Private-for-profit organisations operated over 50 per cent of the aged care homes in Australia and, in 2016, the Australian Institute of Health and Welfare found about half of these had more than 100 places. It is argued that financial viability drove the increase in size.

Australian aged care homes appear to be going against the overseas trend towards smaller living units. For example, the Green House Project in the USA has constructed more than 185 homes each housing 10 – 12 residents. Studies have shown that these residents have an enhanced quality of life without compromising either their clinical care or the cost of running these houses.

In Australia, a 2018 Flinders University study into residents with dementia found that in smaller home-like facilities with up to 15 residents, the dementia residents had a better quality of life (as rated by the residents themselves or family members), 68 per cent lower rate of hospitalisations, 73 per cent lower rate of emergency department presentation and 52 per cent less likely to be exposed to potentially inappropriate medications such as antipsychotics or relaxants often prescribed to residential care residents. The cost of providing care was no higher, and in fact lower in some cases, than in the larger 'institutional' facilities. The World Health Organisation has also supported small home-like residential units stating that they 'hold promise for older people, family members and volunteers who provide care and support'.

Internationally, aged care facilities or nursing homes are moving towards providing care in home-like facilities and promote independence. Such homes generally have greater flexibility in daily routines; for example when residents may get dressed or eat and even opportunity for residents to participate in domestic activities like preparing meals or gardening. Another important aspect was that staff were assigned to units in order to develop relationships between residents and staff as well as continuity of care. Evidence has shown that the physical design of the residential aged care design was important with clusters of smaller living units, access to outdoors and moving away from the 'hospital' style accommodation.

Australia is lagging behind many other countries in offering our elderly alternative models of residential aged care. Is it the large profit driven companies dictating the design to maximise profits or is it governments aiming to minimise costs?

I have recently been speaking to an insider who works at an aged care home operated by one of the large aged care home companies. Staff morale is generally low across all staffing levels. Overworked, underpaid, insufficient staff, lack of basic equipment, lack of support from the organisation and abuse by residents and relatives are some of the areas leading to this low morale. Few aged care workers will speak out about the system as many workers are from overseas and fear losing their employment.

The Australian Government is planning to introduce a star-based system for aged care homes to help people to choose a home when the time comes. Unfortunately, unlike some overseas countries that aim for five stars, the Australian scheme will aim for about 3 stars. How this scheme will be administered, we will have to wait to find out and hopefully it won't be a self-graded scheme or even administered by the current auditing system. At the home that the insider works at, things may seem satisfactory but that is far from the truth. Some basic equipment like hoists and wheel chairs are broken or in short supply, industrial dishwashers are broken or, in one case, the dishwasher only works on one setting. Basic hygiene standards are not followed; for example a lady was getting dressed and lost control of her bowels. Towels were used to clean the floor but no disinfectant was available and it would wait until the cleaners came. Regardless of how clean the staff member was able to clean the floor, germs would be spread through the other areas as people walked on the floor. The hygiene training carers may have received through training at TAFE is in practice not applied. There have been a number of cases reported where aged care homes have prior notification of audits therefore allowing time to get their system in order.

If this home is fairly typical of others where profit seems to be more important than residents' needs and care, then it is little wonder that Covid had such an effect on aged care facilities in some states. It would appear that it has been more by luck than good management that other aged care facilities did not have the outbreaks of Covid that some aged care homes did.

It is not an easy role for the carers. Imagine a resident who, for whatever reason, doesn't want a shower for days at a time or doesn't want to get out of bed. What can a carer do? What would you do if, as a carer, you were asked for an egg for breakfast but the care package that the resident is on does not allow for bacon and eggs only porridge? Again, these are examples of what happens in this particular home. Carers in some areas are run off their feet by some residents continually buzzing for attention often for trivial requests.

Registered nurses seem to be under-represented for the number of carers reporting to them and when there is a complaint, the registered nurses find it far easier to take the side of the resident or family member thus creating friction amongst the staff.

Not all staff members are really suited to working in aged care and some may burn out over a period of time. This can result in some of the stories of 'abuse' that we hear about. One story that I heard relates to a lady being left on the toilet while a staff member went for morning tea. Another story involved a gentleman who wanted to go to the toilet before having lunch. One staff member said that he could 'go in his pants' - but fortunately another staff member came and took him to the toilet. A relative who has a parent in another aged care facility related her disgust that the home limited the number of incontinence pads per day. All residents deserve dignity.

Most staff are extremely dedicated, even going to the extent of buying clothing for residents when the residents' clothes are worn out. How can such a situation occur? Unfortunately, many residents are placed in these aged care facilities and forgotten about by their families. In one area of the home, staff pointed out only two families had visited their relatives in this particular wing of this aged care home in the last 12 months. For many families, it is 'out of sight, out of mind'. Maybe one of the conditions of residency in these aged care homes should be that family members should visit at least once a month. Many of the Asian community still maintain the nucleus family nucleus and if a member has to go into a home, they still maintain regular contact. For others, affluence has allowed us to place our relatives into these aged care facilities often much sooner than may be required.

I have had relatives in aged care homes and I understand that they are not a pleasant place to visit. I ran the gauntlet of moving past chairs of people slumped in their chairs, eyes closed, mouth opened and dribbling. They had nothing to do and no visitors expected but it provided some exercise to move from their room to the lounge area. I would try to take my mother-in-law out once a week to a coffee shop for a piece of cake and a coffee. She would give me two dollars for a coffee and cake, having no idea that a coffee was four dollars fifty but she didn't need to know. She felt good getting out for a coffee and to buy the coffee.

Wake up Australia, we all have a responsibility for aged care. As we age, we have a responsibility to look after ourselves, keep ourselves as fit and mobile as we can. When we reach the stage that we can't, then we must consider our alternatives. Do we rely on our relatives or the aged care facilities? If we go into an aged care facility then our relatives still have an obligation to visit, not just put us into a facility and pretend that we have died. We also can't rely on our government to throw billions of dollars at our aged care problem and expect money to fix the issue.

Australia is to have a rating system to make it easier for older Australians and their families to assess and compare the quality of aged care providers. Unlike overseas 'star' ratings such as the United Kingdom and the USA, Australia has developed a colour-coded bar scale. It has been developed by the Department of Health and the Aged Care Quality and Safety Commission in conjunction with input provided by senior Australians, caregivers, providers and peak bodies. The ratings are expected to show the provider's current position in regards to the most recent performance assessment and any sanctions or non-compliance notices. It will be based solely on the Quality Commission's audits and assessment without taking into account any consumer feedback. Why is there no consumer feedback included; after all, these are the people most affected? Why is past performance over three, five or even ten years not provided?

Not all aged care facilities are government funded but those that are are required to comply with eight Aged Care Quality Standards which reflect the level of care and services the community expects from aged care providers. The eight standards are:

1. Consumer dignity and choice

2. Ongoing assessment and planning

3. Personal care and clinical care

4. Service and support for daily living

5. Organisation's service environment

6. Feedback and complaints

7. Human resources

8. Organisational governance.

As one who had worked in government for almost 20 years and at times developed such standards, I can say that these standards have met the requirements of the bureaucrats but what do they mean in practice? The Australian Government website My Aged Care has a very brief explanation. If you have relatives in aged care or are knowledgeable about aged care, see if you agree with these standards and how they may be assessed.

Australian aged care has had some 20 reports in the last 20 years and recently a Royal Commission. The interim report of the Royal Commission into Aged Care Quality and Safety noted that:

1. It lacks fundamental transparency

2. Very little information is available to the public about the performance of service providers

3. A number of complaints against them are not published

4. A number of assaults in their services are not published

5. A number of staff employed to provide care are not published

6. Participation by providers in the collection of a very limited set of performance indicators only became compulsory on 1 July 2019

7. My Aged Care website "often" doesn't provide "helpful information" about local care providers

8. Older people and their loved ones do not know what to look for when choosing a home.

This last point highlights that education is lacking and easily understandable options are not available not only in aged care facilities but in everything to do with aged care.

The Carnell-Paterson review in 2017 noted a "striking feature" of Australia's aged care system was a lack of reliable, comparable information about quality standards in residential aged care.

Australia does not need to reinvent the wheel. There are good examples from other countries which collect data on hospitalisations, falls, use of antipsychotic medication, urinary tract infections, catheters, hours per day per resident by various staff such as registered nurses, nurses aids, therapists as well as complaints and abuse. Ratings in the United Kingdom cover yearly health inspections over a three year period and focus on deficiencies in such areas as nutrition and dietary needs, residents' rights, nursing services, quality of life and care.

The question needs to be asked; 'How good is the agency that will be undertaking such audits?' There are over 200,000 aged Australians per day in aged care residences relying upon these audits to be conducted fairly and openly.

Thankfully, alternatives to traditional aged care are slowly emerging, including models that maximise independence, promote individual choices and social connectedness. Possibly one of the most talked about options, among friends, is the possibility of them buying into the same apartment block or building their own units on a block of land where they can share the cost of the care services as required.

New Direction Care in Queensland is offering a different community concept for those with complex care needs. Over 6 streets, there is a café, a hairdresser, a corner store and 17 homes each with 7 residents. Residents of a house have similar lifestyles and values and multi-skilled house companions cook meals, do the laundry and provide personal care in consultation with the residents and allied health professionals.

With retirement villages and aged care facilities, one must carefully examine the entry fees, ongoing costs and exit fees. These vary widely and it is worth getting legal and financial advice so that you and your family understand all the fees and charges associated with this style of accommodation.

Many other retirees want to explore Australia and/or the world before settling into either a new home, a retirement village or going back to their family home.

Alternatives to traditional housing concepts

Not everyone is happy with the housing options outlined above and Baby Boomers are looking at other options in retirement. According to an *Australian Financial Review* article, a group of 125 adults and 40 children have purchased a 63 hectare site on the NSW Central Coast and plan to build 110 low-footprint dwellings and develop a multi-generational community.

Others are going to the other extreme and exploring tiny houses, sometimes being built in residential backyards. To conform to some council requirements, they are being built on a wheeled base, similar to a caravan, and are not connected to sewerage. However not all councils approve of the concept which could allow the tiny house to be transported to another site.

There are a number of other options being proposed including what is basically a modified rooming house. From the street, they look like a normal house but inside there may be 4-6 units. Each unit has its own kitchenette, en-suite, space for a bed and lounge area within a self-contained area. The units all have access from a common recreational area and there may be one car space for a communally-owned car. They are designed to provide cheap accommodation to owner-occupiers or tenants.

Councils around Australia are not keeping pace with the options that developers are proposing.

Joining the grey nomads

For many, retirement is the chance to buy a 4WD vehicle and a caravan or a recreation vehicle like a Winnebago. They can travel to remote parts of Australia for extended periods ranging from a few months to a few years. Part of the appeal of becoming a grey nomad is the desire to meet other retirees, share in the adventures and develop new friendships. For some, this brings back childhood memories of going caravanning with their parents. It was not so much a road trip but a trip down to the coast, at the same time each year, camping on the same site year after year and surrounded by the same families that would also do the same thing each year. Depending upon the retiree's employment background, some are able to get some part-time work along the way which helps stretch the budget while travelling.

When preparing a budget for your travels, be realistic and always have a contingency. Fuel will always be far more expensive than you expect and towing a caravan will also use more fuel. Hotels in some regional areas offer free overnight camping areas in return for having a beer or two and a dinner at the pub.

If you are contemplating such a lifestyle, do not wait until retirement to go out and buy that 4WD and the caravan or the mobile home. Purchase the vehicle a few years before retirement and take small trips in order to get the feel of the vehicle and towing the caravan. Plan where you would like to visit and then make sure that your vehicle and caravan are appropriate for the trip.

I have personally worked in some of the communities in the Northern Peninsula Area of Queensland and seen many travellers having an extended holiday in a township like Bamaga because their vehicles or caravan were not suited to the conditions that they encountered. It can be time consuming and costly to have replacement parts transported to isolated regions of Australia when vehicles break down. Unsealed corrugated roads take their toll on vehicles in the most unexpected ways.

House-sitting

House-sitting is not a widely known exercise. A number of retirees that we know have house-sat both in Australia and overseas. The periods for house-sitting seem to vary widely from a couple of weeks to a year. Sitters enjoy rent-free accommodation in return for looking after the garden and pets although this differs from house to house. One retiree I heard of who house-sat for about eight months did have to look after a dog but the house owners had a gardener who came in every couple of weeks.

The benefit to the house owner is that their pets can stay in familiar surroundings at home saving on the cost of kennels and the house is occupied thus providing some security while the owners are away.

There are a number of companies in Australia that match a potential house-sitter with the owner of the house.

Similar house-sitting can occur in many countries around the world. This can provide a good base for exploring a particular area and to live like a local.

House swap

Also known as house exchange, it is a little different from the house-sitting discussed above. With a house swap, you select the area of the world that you would like to visit, then advertise your house and negotiate with people who would like to live in your house. Each home-owner continues to pay rates, insurance and maintenance while they are away. You will need to inform your insurance company of the proposed arrangement but most companies seem happy to have the house occupied rather than being vacant for an extended period of time.

The advantage, apart from saving money, is that you have a home atmosphere with full cooking facilities and, depending on the arrangements, a car at your disposal. The house is an ideal base from which you can explore other parts of the country or even other countries without taking large suitcases on each trip.

Think outside the box

I read an interesting article where an American couple sold their house and lived in hotels operated by the Hilton chain. A couple of years ago, a friend of mine did a similar thing. A single guy, retired from the defence forces and undertaking part-time locum work, he liked travelling. His house in Sydney was under-utilised so, after some consideration, he gave away most of his worldly possessions and sold his house.

Today, he travels the world staying in 5-star hotels and believes that he is financially better off. No longer does he have to consider the following in his budget:

- Council rates
- Water rates
- House insurance
- Contents insurance
- Repairs and maintenance
- Interest repayments
- Body Corporate fees
- Electricity
- Internet
- Cleaning
- Gardening
- Security
- Gym membership

- Pool maintenance
- Parking
- Car registration
- Car insurance
- Replacing furniture or white goods

Nowadays, he lives where he wants – a hotel by the beach, in the country or in the centre of any of the great cities of the world. Hotel membership may provide free breakfasts, morning and afternoon teas and canapes in the evening in the executive lounge. He is also likely to receive free internet, cable TV and free local or interstate phone calls. As a guest of the hotel he receives daily housekeeping and laundry services, access to a pool, gym, security, and beautiful hotel gardens in prime locations. If he is unsure where to go for that special evening meal or needs a special present, then he contacts the hotel concierge.

If you stay with one or two particular hotel chains, you will quickly build up points for free nights and your status with the hotel may allow early check-in and late check-outs plus room upgrades.

So there are many options to consider in planning where and how you may live in retirement. There is no one-fits-all. The accommodation, or combinations of accommodation that you choose, is as individual as you are but remember to take a long-term view.

Do not sell the family home too quickly. Remember the six-year rule of the Australian Taxation Office and talk with your accountant before experimenting with living options.

Living alone

Some people are happy (and have chosen) to live alone. Unfortunately, for others who have lived together for many years, living alone is not a desirable situation. It is sensible to consider what your life might be like alone. What things might have to change? What are the practicalities of living alone? What additional things would you have to do around the house? Some people enjoy living on their own but there is a big difference between living on your own while working and living on your own in retirement. Work provides a structure to your day, with friends and colleagues to mix with and maybe go out with socially. In retirement, you have to add some structure to your life and be proactive in retaining friendships.

As we have mentioned previously, divorce is occurring more frequently in the age group over 50 so we may find ourselves home alone. The second reason that we may find ourselves living alone is through a serious and maybe long-term illness of our partner such as dementia or Alzheimer's disease. The third potential reason for living alone is through the death of a partner. Cruelly, plans that you have made together for the next 20 years will seem pointless. Humans, generally, crave companionship so living alone can lead to a danger of becoming self-absorbed. Some people may want independence but independence should not be confused with isolation. Independence is good, isolation is not.

If living alone is thrust upon you, you need to talk with family and friends over a period of time to see what you may do. Do you remain in your house? Do you consider some live-in help or co-habit with someone else? Do you sell and move in with one of your children or into a retirement village? Can you build a granny flat and move into that while renting out the main house? Are there any pension considerations and what timeframes are there to consider?

In summary, whether as a couple or an individual, the choice of where you live is important for a number of reasons:

1. Many memories associated with your children
2. Maintaining contact and friendships with long term neighbours
3. Familiarity with services in the area, for example public transport

The decision of where you live is ultimately yours.

A good home base may be important if you wish to travel.

Chapter 9

Travel in style

The journey, not the arrival, matters.

TS Eliot

"Twenty years from now, you will be more disappointed by the things that you didn't do than by the ones you did do. So throw off the bowlines. Sail away from the safe harbour. Catch the tradewinds in your sails. Explore. Dream. Discover."

Sarah Frances Brown

For many, travel has long been associated with retirement both as a sign of commencing retirement and as an activity in retirement. Today, retirement still means travel as you are no longer bound by taking your annual leave at a certain time each year. But, like many other aspects, potential retirees seeking to travel need to be preparing and planning for whatever travel they are going to undertake. For the more adventurous and healthy who plan to hike or bike ride around certain parts of the world, this may mean getting a little fitter. For others, it might mean finding a cruise or tour company that will organise everything. Whatever your travel plans are, your plans should involve research. This is good for your brain but it is good to understand the countries you are visiting; the history, the customs, and the people. It will make for a more rewarding trip.

Retirement is a great time to take advantage of last-minute deals that come up with airlines and cruises. Imagine opening the newspaper or turning on the television and see a fantastic trip being offered, leaving in two weeks' time. How great to have the freedom, to be able to book that cruise or that holiday (after checking your diary for any other engagements). For those who want to be more organised, there are also good deals to be made by booking well in advance.

If work or holidays involve travel then there are things that you need to be doing, prior to retirement, in order to take advantage of airline and hotel benefits. We will explore these in more detail later in this chapter.

Australia

For a few decades, grey nomads have taken to the roads of Australia to visit places that, for many, they have had on their bucket list for many years. Others might be just exploring. Australia is a big country with diverse weather conditions so careful planning is important.

It is important to understand that heading to the northern parts of Australia during the summer months will mean hot weather, storms and the potential for cyclones and floods. If travelling during these times, be prepared for delays. After the wet, semi-trailers are likely to have been the first vehicles through, taking supplies to remote towns. Unless the local council has been through with a grader, the semi-trailers are likely to have disturbed the road surface making the roads almost impassable, particularly for a caravan.

All roads are not the same, even those with a bitumen surface; some are narrow with little room on the side of the roads to pull over or stop. Be aware of high wind areas particularly if towing a caravan. When it comes to some of the development roads, these can be very frustrating for novices driving on corrugations with bulldust. Be prepared to take your time, find the right speed that will make the corrugations more bearable, and stick to that speed limit. This speed limit may well be below the sign-posted speed limit.

Prepare your vehicle for the areas that you plan to visit. This may involve taking extra tyres or even a satellite phone.

For an interesting blog on outback travels, take a look at *Bulldust and Back Roads* particularly if you plan to travel with a dog. James and Trinity travel with Mr Dog, so look for dog friendly locations to camp.

Australia is a great and diversified country with thousands and thousands of kilometres to explore. Be aware of potential dangers such as kangaroos, cattle, wild horses and camels – not forgetting other road users, especially road trains. If you see a road train coming towards you or coming up behind you, pull over to the side of the road and allow them the full width of the road. The last trailer can have a fair amount of sway so give them room. When you travel, try to drive between 8am and 4pm to avoid animals like kangaroos looking for food. Always be on the lookout for overnight road kills as these can damage your vehicle or cause you to swerve.

Before any long trip, have your vehicle serviced and make sure you have, and know how to operate, any safety equipment. If it is a new vehicle, do some shorter trips to get acquainted with it. If a new 4WD has been purchased, or a caravan added, why not consider some of the courses available for caravanning or four wheel driving?

Overseas travel

Australians young and old are great travellers so it is not uncommon when travelling to come across fellow Australians, sometimes in remote places. Many Australians have a bucket list of overseas destinations to visit, some while working but others reserved for retirement when there are not the time constraints of employment.

To travel overseas we have only two choices – air or sea. The choice will be partly dictated by the holiday being planned. Whichever one you choose, there are ways of enjoying benefits that most people are not aware of…..

Firstly, your most valuable document is your passport. Your passport is necessary for booking overseas holidays and as a means of identification at airports and hotels. It is essential to keep it safe and secure at all times. If it is lost or stolen, contact the nearest Australian Embassy or Australian Consulate. The important thing with passports is that, although they may technically have a 10-year life, the reality is that for many countries you are required to have between three and six months validity remaining on your passport. It is important to check the passport requirements for each country that is on your itinerary to ensure you have the minimum length of time remaining on your passport. Being refused entry to a particular country due to not having the minimum time prior to expiry of your passport could have major implications for the remainder of the holiday. A refusal of entry in one country could result in you not being able to complete your holiday. If you are able to continue, there are likely to be additional costs involved with cancelled or rearranged flights, hotels and sightseeing tours.

Some countries require Australians to obtain visas either prior to departing Australia or at immigration prior to entering the country. Again, know the requirements of the countries that you are visiting and allow sufficient time for the visa to be obtained. Sometimes, this may involve sending your passport and an application to another city such as Canberra.

A number of years ago, I was going to visit France but instead of obtaining a visa in Australia, I planned to obtain one from the French Embassy in London. I had to join the queue, in the rain, outside the French Embassy with no certainty that I would be successful in getting a visa on the first attempt. A couple of people that I spoke to, while I waited, had been in the queue the previous day. They had to return because the embassy closed the doors at a certain time regardless of how many people were waiting.

Depending on where you are travelling to, it is important to check what vaccinations, if any, are required. If vaccinations are required, allow sufficient time to obtain all the vaccination doses required. There may be a delay of maybe 14 days between the first dose of the vaccine and the second. Make sure that the vaccination card is completed by the doctor and that it is packed with your passport.

Also make sure that you are aware of all requirements of countries that you may visit or transit through. In October 2018, the United Arab Emirates introduced a requirement that all travellers had to submit a list of all prescription and non-prescription medications to the Ministry of Health prior to travel. In 2019, an Australian couple were detained for a few months in Iran for having flown a drone without a permit.

For many Australians travelling overseas, tipping can become a bit of an issue. Before any travel, understand the requirements for tipping in any country you plan to visit. If you tip in Australia, it is an acknowledgement of good food and good service. In countries like the USA, tips form part of a person's income and are often unrelated to the quality of service. You would not visit the USA without many $1.00 notes and that is just to cover the tipping required between the airport and your hotel room. In the USA, tipping is no longer 10 per cent of the bill; that rule is out of date. In some countries, like Japan, tipping even to acknowledge good service is frowned upon. Research the countries you plan to visit and go prepared both mentally and with appropriate small denominations of money for tips.

Airlines

There are three main global airline alliances:

1. One World with members such as Qantas, British Airways, Cathay Pacific, Emirates and American Airlines
2. Star Alliances with members such as Air New Zealand, Singapore Airlines and Thai Airways.
3. Sky Team with members such as Aeroflot, Air France, Garuda Indonesia, Korean Air and United Airlines.

There are also some other airlines that are not part of these three alliances but have relationships with other airlines. For example, Etihad has relationships with Air Canada and Air France, Qantas has relationships with Fiji Airways and Aer Lingus and Alaskan Airlines has relationships with Qantas, Delta Airlines and Emirates.

These relationships can change over time and can cut across some alliances. For example, Delta Airlines is a member of Sky Team whereas Qantas and Emirates are One World but all three have a relationship with Alaskan Airlines. Recently, the alliance between Virgin Australia and Air New Zealand ended. Qantas and Air New Zealand have now formed a new alliance.

This is far from an exhaustive list of airlines and their alliances and relationships. So how do you consider which airline or alliance might be best for you?

Firstly you need to consider your flying history and flying future. Who have you flown with in the past and which countries are you likely to visit in the future? Do you currently have any frequent flyer memberships with any airlines? Being a resident of Australia, we often just think of flying either Qantas or Virgin Australia but the alliances and relationships that airlines have opens up a whole new world of airlines you can fly with.

One trip that I did in December 2014 involved booking my flights through American Airlines. I was escorted through the terminal at Heathrow London to the British Airways first class lounge before travelling in the front of a Qantas plane. I had a layover in Dubai and access to the Emirates first class lounge then continued back to Australia, on Qantas, again as a first class passenger. It was an absolutely unbelievable trip and at a cost of about one fifth of a normal first class ticket. Since then, I have undertaken other overseas flights involving aircraft of different carriers but of the same alliance. This is available through a code-sharing arrangement that the airline has with other airlines.

One of the advantages of retirees is flexibility and, with airlines, flexibility needs to be your friend. There are huge savings to be made if you are flexible with the dates that you travel. Sometimes it may be only a couple of days and, at other times it may be a week or a month. Tuesday, Wednesday and Saturday are normally cheaper days to fly and the dearest period to book a flight is around one or two weeks before departure. Some of the best times to book airfares are between 21-60 days before departure. There can be variations to these timeframes; for example, seasons and local events. Anyone in Australia is well aware that the airlines rapidly increase the price of airfares for the various football grand finals. For travelling overseas there are also peak, shoulder and off-peak seasons and, during the peak periods, airfares are the most expensive and hardest to acquire.

Flying in Australia is expensive due to government charges and fuel surcharges but not all airlines have similar charges, particularly in regard to the fuel surcharge. You can save hundreds of dollars depending upon the airport that you fly into and out of. For example, it is cheaper to fly into Manchester England or an airport in Paris than it is into Heathrow in London. It may mean a change of travel plans and a small extra cost of getting from Manchester or Paris to London or vice versa but the cost saving is worth considering. Recently, the United Kingdom (UK) introduced a departure tax of approximately $315 that is applied to any international flights departing UK airports.

Regardless of whether you are in first class, business, premium economy or economy, not all seats are the same. Some are located near the galley or the toilets, others may have extra legroom due to emergency exits and, in some cases, a window seat may have no window due to the structural requirements of the plane. There is an app called SeatGuru that helps identify the good from the bad seats. Past passengers have provided reviews of the seat locations so it is a useful website. You may ask your travel agent or the check-in staff for a particular seat or to change an allocated seat depending on what you find on SeatGuru. Unfortunately, it cannot help with whom you may be seated next to!

If you travel frequently, or even one return trip to Europe or America, you will accumulate a significant number of points, miles or status credits depending upon the airline flown and the frequent flyer scheme. Some airlines allocate points or miles based on the miles flown but the more common method now is based on the revenue, that is, dollars spent. Some airlines like Qantas earn both points and status credits per flight. The points can be used to redeem flights, to upgrade a flight or to purchase merchandise whereas earning a certain number of status credits within a 12-month period may lead to silver, gold, platinum or platinum one status. The greater status you achieve, the more benefits can be enjoyed such as priority check-in and seat selection. Although the status credit requirement is reset at the anniversary of membership, the status credits continue to accumulate towards lifetime silver and then lifetime gold for Qantas. Qantas recently introduced a lifetime platinum level but the sky high requirements are unrealistic for most travellers. Frequent flyers that I know are crediting their points and status to British Airways where achieving Lifetime Platinum is more achievable. Other airlines have similar schemes.

Some airlines will allow frequent flyer members to purchase points or miles, sometimes at a discount, and this can be an attractive method for booking flights as I did with my American Airline flight in 2014. Qantas does not allow members to purchase points as some other airlines do but it will allow members to top up their points if they fall short of the points required for a particular trip. No points or status credits are earned when a member flies on a flight paid for with points or miles. Airlines publish tables on their website showing the number of points or miles required for particular flights. My flight in 2014 from London to Melbourne in first class, then Melbourne to Brisbane in business class, cost 80,000 miles plus some government charges. I did have to be a little flexible with dates and came back to Australia about three days ahead of my planned return.

For those who enjoy flying and want status with an airline, some frequent flyer members undertake what is known as 'status run'. The sole purpose of a status run is to accumulate the miles, points or status credit needed when short of status credits to maintain a current membership level or achieve a higher status. The following is not a status run that would be used but you could fly from Brisbane to Melbourne then to Auckland before flying back to Sydney and on to Cairns and finally back to Brisbane. Such a trip could be done in a couple of days depending on the flights available. However, there is little time for sightseeing.

Mistaken fares

Occasionally, airlines will publish fares that are incorrect. Some travellers with a good knowledge of fares and the time to travel book these fares during the short window of opportunity before the airline realises the mistake. It is at the discretion of the airlines as to whether they will honour the mistaken fare that has been booked.

In early January 2019, Air New Zealand published a round trip business class between Chicago and Australia for under $1500. A couple of days later, Air New Zealand honoured the bookings for the lucky few that had seen the fare and booked. It was for travel between 12 January and 30 November 2019. Air New Zealand provided a non-stop flight from Chicago to Auckland then onto Brisbane, Sydney or Melbourne or with United Airlines through Los Angeles or San Francisco to Australia.

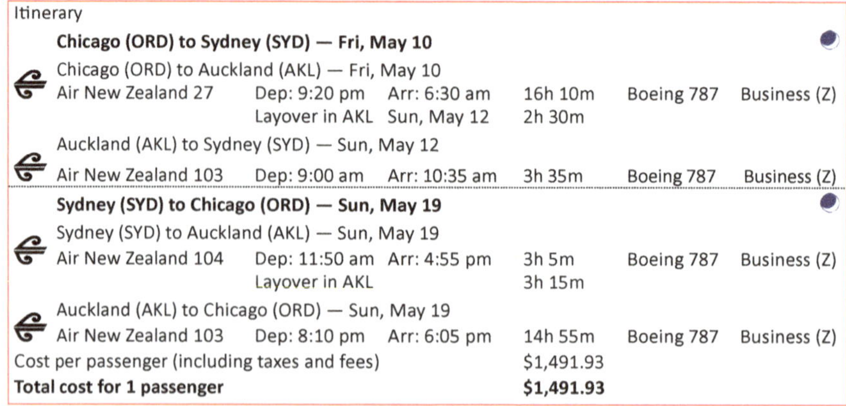

Itinerary

Chicago (ORD) to Sydney (SYD) — Fri, May 10

Chicago (ORD) to Auckland (AKL) — Fri, May 10

| Air New Zealand 27 | Dep: 9:20 pm | Arr: 6:30 am | 16h 10m | Boeing 787 | Business (Z) |
| | Layover in AKL | Sun, May 12 | 2h 30m | | |

Auckland (AKL) to Sydney (SYD) — Sun, May 12

| Air New Zealand 103 | Dep: 9:00 am | Arr: 10:35 am | 3h 35m | Boeing 787 | Business (Z) |

Sydney (SYD) to Chicago (ORD) — Sun, May 19

Sydney (SYD) to Auckland (AKL) — Sun, May 19

| Air New Zealand 104 | Dep: 11:50 am | Arr: 4:55 pm | 3h 5m | Boeing 787 | Business (Z) |
| | Layover in AKL | | 3h 15m | | |

Auckland (AKL) to Chicago (ORD) — Sun, May 19

| Air New Zealand 103 | Dep: 8:10 pm | Arr: 6:05 pm | 14h 55m | Boeing 787 | Business (Z) |

Cost per passenger (including taxes and fees) $1,491.93
Total cost for 1 passenger **$1,491.93**

Example fare provided by OMAAT

In late December 2018, Cathay Pacific published insane business and first class fares for travel between Vietnam and Canada for $988 return and Vietnam and United States of America for $1445 return.

The mistaken fares were quickly removed but for those that had managed to book, Cathay Pacific honoured the fares.

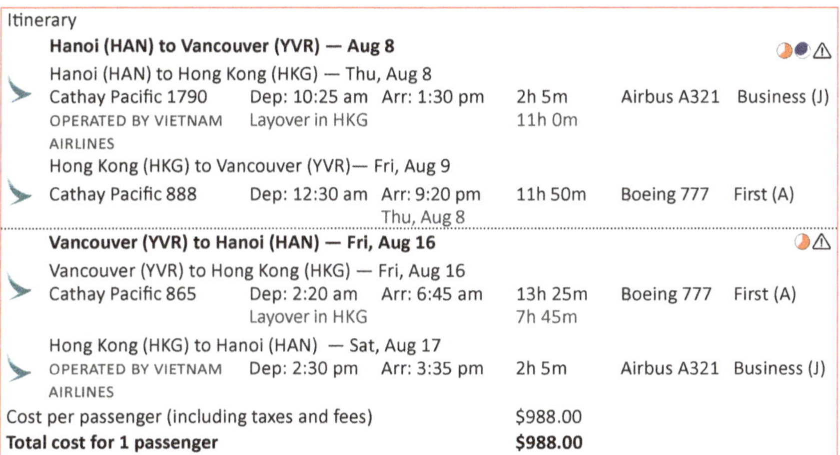

Example fares provided by OMAAT.

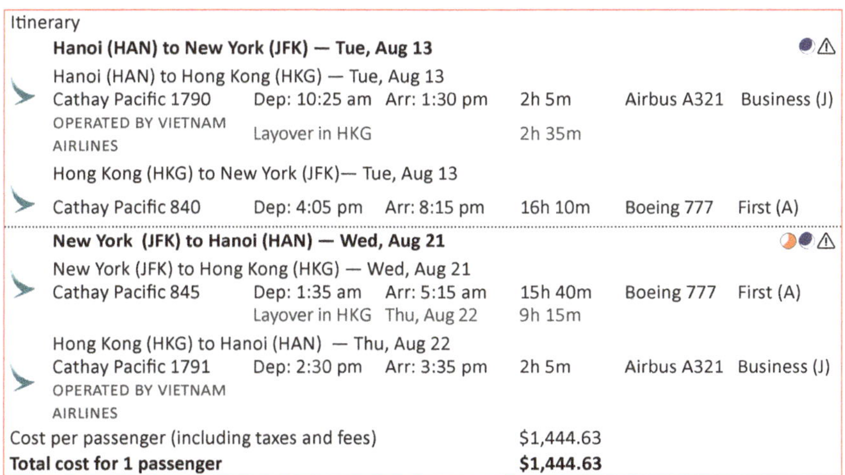

Other examples were Hanoi to Washington DC business class return for $1560 and first class on the same route for $1812 return. A normal first class return fare would be around $15,000.

It should be noted that mistaken fares are rare and not all airlines will honour them. A fare on 5 January 2019 involved a flight from Kuala Lumpur to Dubai. Bookings were made through Malaysian Airlines on a flight operated by Emirates. The same fare was not offered on Emirates. The tickets that were issued at the mistaken fare were cancelled, and money refunded, without the customers being notified.

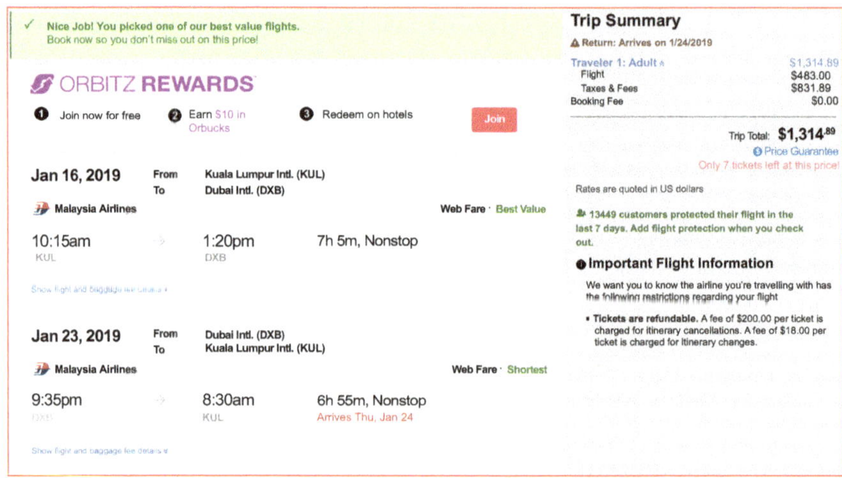

Note the taxes and fees compared to the actual flight cost.

It is acknowledged that these destinations may not be on your bucket list but with some planning around these fares, a traveller could construct an interesting holiday, flying with good airlines and on nice aircraft.

Asia to Europe

We have already mentioned the fuel surcharges and other airport fees that make flying from Australia expensive. Have you considered flying out of Asia? As the following fares show, you can fly business class from Asia at a fraction of the cost of flying from Australia even allowing for a flight from Australia to Asia. Again, if you are flexible, you can fly into some great European cities and then construct your holiday from these cities.

In the following examples, Manila has been selected as the Asian city from which the airlines will fly to Europe. You will need to book a return flight from Australia to Manila on Qantas, Philippine Airlines or another airline and maybe have a day in Manila on the way over and again on the way back. This should allow for any flight delays and lessen your chance of missing the connecting flight.

You could use your frequent flyer points from other travel to pay for your return flights to Asia.

The following example is a return business class flight on Etihad Airways from Manila to Rome via Abu Dhabi. The cost is approximately A$2570.00.

The Etihad sale ended 30 October 2019 and travel had to be commenced from Manila by 31 August 2020. Etihad allows a free stopover in Abu Dhabi in both directions.

Such a return trip between Manila and Rome would earn approximately 400 status credits and about 16,200 Velocity points.

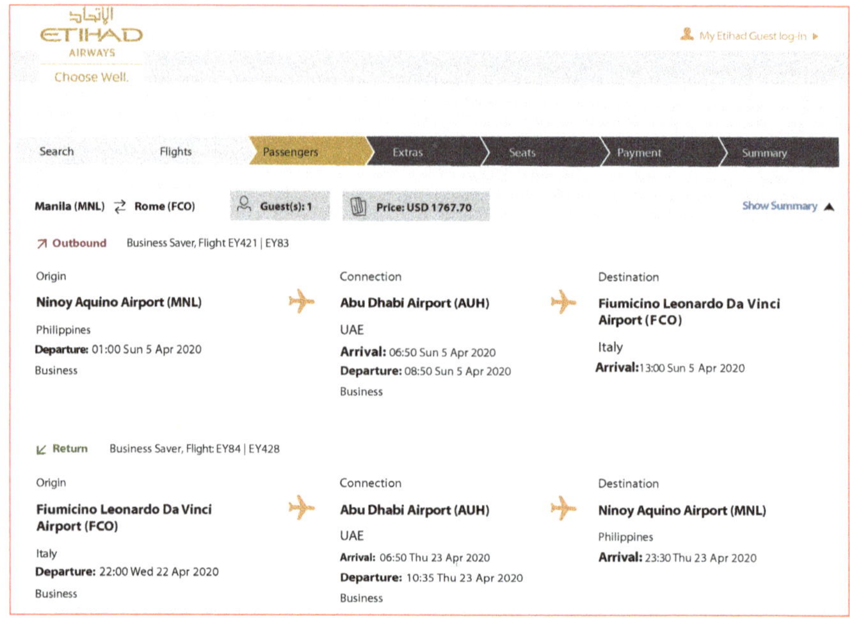

A second example is travelling on Qatar Airways, again between Manila and Rome.

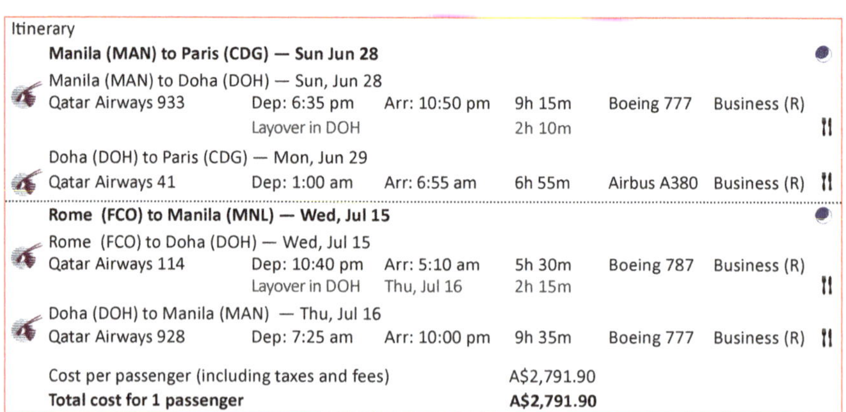

Itinerary

Manila (MAN) to Paris (CDG) — Sun Jun 28

Manila (MAN) to Doha (DOH) — Sun, Jun 28

| Qatar Airways 933 | Dep: 6:35 pm | Arr: 10:50 pm | 9h 15m | Boeing 777 | Business (R) |
| | Layover in DOH | | 2h 10m | | |

Doha (DOH) to Paris (CDG) — Mon, Jun 29

| Qatar Airways 41 | Dep: 1:00 am | Arr: 6:55 am | 6h 55m | Airbus A380 | Business (R) |

Rome (FCO) to Manila (MNL) — Wed, Jul 15

Rome (FCO) to Doha (DOH) — Wed, Jul 15

| Qatar Airways 114 | Dep: 10:40 pm | Arr: 5:10 am | 5h 30m | Boeing 787 | Business (R) |
| | Layover in DOH | Thu, Jul 16 | 2h 15m | | |

Doha (DOH) to Manila (MAN) — Thu, Jul 16

| Qatar Airways 928 | Dep: 7:25 am | Arr: 10:00 pm | 9h 35m | Boeing 777 | Business (R) |

| Cost per passenger (including taxes and fees) | A$2,791.90 |
| **Total cost for 1 passenger** | **A$2,791.90** |

The sale ended 29 October 2019 and travel had to commence by 31 August 2020. If you are a member of Qantas Frequent Flyer, you could earn approximately 14,500 points plus 320 status credits. If you are a member of another One World airline frequent flyer scheme, you could credit the flights towards that airline's scheme.

To illustrate that some flexibility is required, Emirates also had business class fares but departed from Clark International Airport, about three hours drive from Manila. The destination was Milan, Italy, via Dubai. The return airport was Cebu.

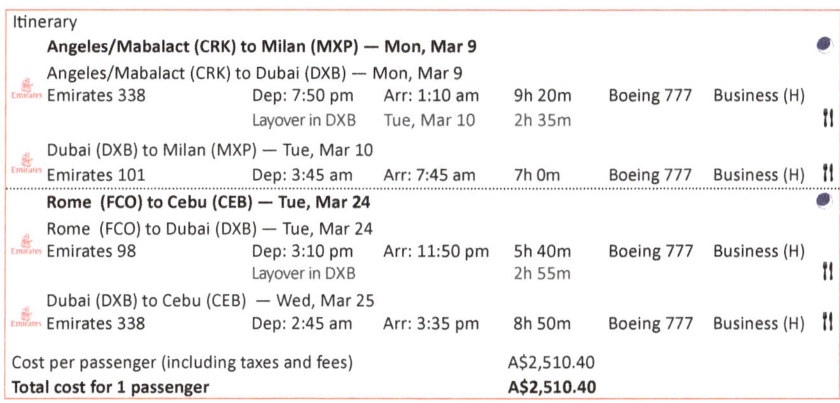

Itinerary						
Angeles/Mabalact (CRK) to Milan (MXP) — Mon, Mar 9						
Angeles/Mabalact (CRK) to Dubai (DXB) — Mon, Mar 9						
Emirates 338	Dep: 7:50 pm	Arr: 1:10 am	9h 20m	Boeing 777	Business (H)	
	Layover in DXB	Tue, Mar 10	2h 35m			
Dubai (DXB) to Milan (MXP) — Tue, Mar 10						
Emirates 101	Dep: 3:45 am	Arr: 7:45 am	7h 0m	Boeing 777	Business (H)	
Rome (FCO) to Cebu (CEB) — Tue, Mar 24						
Rome (FCO) to Dubai (DXB) — Tue, Mar 24						
Emirates 98	Dep: 3:10 pm	Arr: 11:50 pm	5h 40m	Boeing 777	Business (H)	
	Layover in DXB		2h 55m			
Dubai (DXB) to Cebu (CEB) — Wed, Mar 25						
Emirates 338	Dep: 2:45 am	Arr: 3:35 pm	8h 50m	Boeing 777	Business (H)	
Cost per passenger (including taxes and fees)			A$2,510.40			
Total cost for 1 passenger			**A$2,510.40**			

Emirates is a member of One World alliance so the flights again could be credited to your Qantas Frequent Flyer scheme or remain with Emirates if you plan to fly frequently with Emirates.

These are examples of some of the fares available. There are also fares available from destinations in Indonesia, Malaysia, Thailand and Sri Lanka.

There are a variety of airlines that fly from Asia to Europe including Gulf Air, KLM, Oman Air and Turkish Airlines.

Round The World and Multi-city fares

With a Round The World fare, you basically circumnavigate the globe by going in one continuous direction, either east or west. Round The World fares are offered by airline alliances such as One World, Star Alliance and Sky Team. Each alliance has different rules: for example One World alliance stipulates a minimum of four continents; you can travel in any direction within a continental zone, and have up to 16 sectors plus 2 stopovers. Travelling with the alliances means that you can earn valuable frequent flyer points while travelling on different airlines within the alliance. Most routes follow the major tourist destinations but there is normally an opportunity to undertake side trips.

Round The World fares are typically fixed price and don't fluctuate with travel in peak or off-peak seasons.

Known by a number of names such as Multi-city, Multi-destination or Multi-stop tickets, the fares allow for 3 or more flights covering 2 or more world zones. Normally there is a maximum of 12 sectors and no requirement to go in one direction.

Sometimes Round The World fares are cheaper than a direct flight or Multi-city fares – but not always. It depends partly on the number of flights and your destinations. Recently, I looked at travelling to Athens using a One World alliance carrier. With one carrier, I would fly to London then back to Athens, on another I would fly to Dubai then to Athens but the cheaper option was to book a Round The World trip which included Athens as one of the destinations.

Round The World and Multi-city fares can be a great way to sample different parts of the world. If you like a destination then add it to your bucket list of places to visit in more depth.

Stopovers and layovers

If you plan to do a lot of travelling, it is likely that you will hear these terms, sometimes incorrectly used.

A layover is basically the time waiting for a connecting flight. For example you may be flying from Brisbane to Adelaide via Melbourne. You fly from Brisbane to Melbourne then are required to change planes to fly from Melbourne to Adelaide, possibly with a 2-hour layover between one flight and the next. For domestic air travel, a layover is generally less than 4 hours but, for international travel, it can be just under 24 hours. Layovers do not have a significant impact for domestic travel but if you had a layover on an international flight of, say 14 hours, and mostly during daylight hours, it may give you the opportunity to have a quick tour of the city.

Stopovers are more likely to occur on international flights. For example, if you were flying from Sydney to London via Dubai, you may be able to have a stopover for a day or two in Dubai before continuing your journey to London.

Some airlines promote stopovers at no additional cost. Some airline routes may not allow stopovers but you may be able to have a long layover during which time you may be able to explore the city.

Visa requirements may affect layover and stopover plans so you would need to check the country's requirements.

Credit cards, shopping and airline points
Some people can become obsessive about using their credit cards to purchase goods or shop at certain stores in order to obtain shopping or airline points.

Over the years there has been much research undertaken to show how much money needed to be spent to obtain a rewards airline flight and other rewards. Generally, it is not worth the effort. If points are accumulated in the course of everyday shopping, then it is a bonus.

It is also worth considering the best use of these points. For example, do you credit your points to an airline or accumulate them with a particular store in order to get maybe $10 off your shopping bill? Each person will value the points differently; some will be happy to let the points accumulate over many months or years for an airline reward while others may like a more instant gratification with $10 off the shopping bill once the required number of points has been reached.

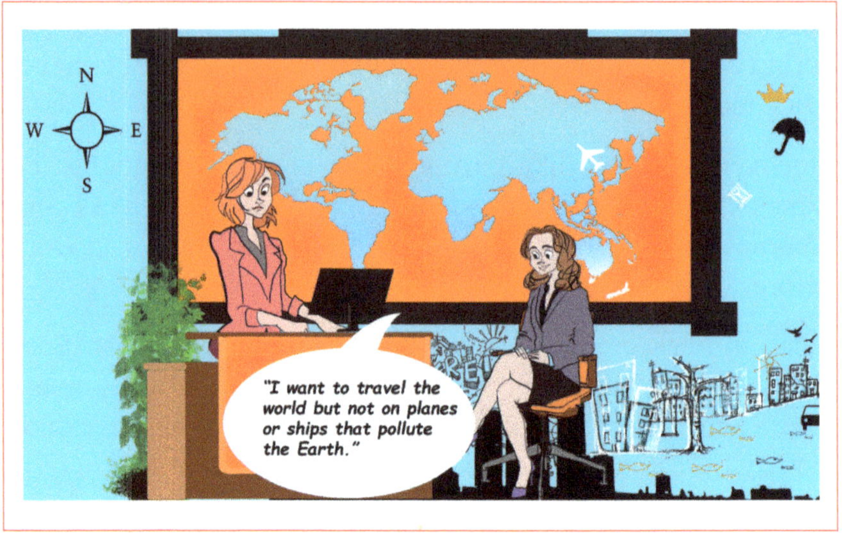

Cruises

The cruise market in Australia has dramatically increased in the past decade and some retirees may have visions of sailing out of Sydney Heads to signify the end of their working career.

For the savvy cruiser, it is no longer a matter of 'which ship do you like?' It is a matter of where you are likely to cruise to and from and what cruise line covers most of these destinations. Cruises range from a few days to round the world cruises of over 100 days.

As with airlines, the cruise lines also have loyalty programs ranging from some basic benefits to free seven-day cruises. Most cruise lines have five or six loyalty levels based on the number of cruise nights you have spent while a couple of other loyalty packages take into account the cabin and other on board purchases such as spa treatments. So it is similar to the revenue-based models that the airlines use.

The benefits after a cruise or two seem fairly paltry – a free bottle of water or a free scoop of gelato to free drink packages, priority disembarkation, laundry services or free internet. It is dependent upon the cruise line as the passenger progresses through the loyalty ranks.

Some cruise lines have restrictions on children under 18 so, if you are cruising without children, then you are catered for. Other cruise lines have a number of formal dining evenings per cruise where a black suit and tie or tuxedo for the gentlemen and evening gown for the ladies is a minimal requirement.

Train travel

Train travel can be a great way to see the countryside. Some railways with high speed trains in countries like Germany and Japan pride themselves on their punctuality for departure and arriving on schedule.

Depending on the distance to be travelled, trains can be a timely method of traversing the country. Trains can be a good alternative to flying when you consider the total time required for flying such as getting to the airport, time required for check-in prior to departure as well as the flight time. There may be little difference in cost due to the many low-cost airlines, particularly in Europe, but one other advantage over airlines is baggage. Generally there are fewer weight restrictions on baggage that you can take on the trains compared with airlines, particularly the low-cost airlines.

Another nice way to get from point A to point B, particularly if time is limited, is to travel overnight on a train. It is normally cheaper to have a sleeper than it is to rent a hotel room and you can travel a few hundred kilometres while you sleep. If there is a border crossing, the train staff may take your passport so that you can have an uninterrupted sleep.

There are some great train journeys around the world like the Orient Express, The Rocky Mountaineer, The Ghan, The Trans-Siberian railway. Why not add a couple to your bucket list?

There can be some great train passes for travel in Europe and Japan for example. Always confirm the requirements for purchasing and use in advance as many are required to be purchased prior to leaving Australia. The Japanese railway allows you to purchase a train pass within three months of arriving in Japan. On arrival in Japan your passport needs to be stamped to show that you are a visitor and the pass allows unlimited use on many of the railways of Japan including the high-speed trains for a consecutive number of days from when first used. There are some restrictions; for example the pass is not for use on privately owned train lines.

Trains can be a very convenient way to arrive in a city as most major train stations are located towards the city centre and if you have booked accommodation nearby, then it may be a short walk to the hotel.

Tour groups

Tour groups can be a great way to meet people and build long-term friendships. It is also a way to visit countries that you may feel uncomfortable visiting as an individual due to language barriers or safety concerns. For some trips, tour groups are the only way to visit certain areas such as the Antarctic. It is also a good way to understand the history of the region and possibly see items of interest that an independent traveller would not see. One tour that I did in Egypt included a side trip up part of the Nile River to a Nubian village to visit relatives of our tour guide. In Egypt, the government takes tourist safety very seriously following a major incident a number of years ago and each tour group has tourist police accompanying the group. Buses are checked before tourists board and there is increased security at the hotels used by the tour groups.

As we mentioned previously with airlines, understanding luggage requirements for tours is very important. As well as weight restrictions, many companies will have a restriction on hard-case bags and a preference for soft luggage. If there is light plane travel involved, there could be further weight restrictions, possibly down to about 15 kilograms per person.

Yes, loyalty is rewarded with tour groups as well and the rewards vary. It may be a $100 per person discount off your second trip, increasing to $300 per person for six or more group holidays, while for others it may be a $2200 – $2500 discount towards the tenth booking. Another company offers a complimentary gift after you return from the second trip but also up to a five per cent discount off certain trips. Another program has changed in 2018 to a revenue base for the rewards, claiming a benefit to their customers.

Many of the so-called rewards like newsletters are what you would expect from any company and, for some of the more lucrative discounts, you would have to wait a number of years and have spent a large sum of money to achieve such rewards. Remember also that a number of companies already offer discounts for early bookings.

Many tour groups have different loyalty levels like silver, gold, platinum and diamond, each level based on the number of trips undertaken. Some companies specify a certain number of days for a trip to qualify towards the loyalty program.

There is no cost to join most loyalty programs so why not join? It is important not to expect any fantastic rewards despite having spent what could be many thousands of dollars over ten tours.

Companies offering more immediate rewards, particularly practical rewards of luggage, might be more inviting.

Interestingly, back in the 1970s and 1980s, you would receive a quality travel wallet and luggage tags when you received your travel documents. Today, you have to become a member and undertake one trip with some tour companies before you receive your prized travel wallet and luggage tags.

Accommodation

While travelling, you now have a wide range of choices when it comes to accommodation such as hotels, bed and breakfast residences, youth hostels, and Airbnb to name a few.

Airbnb/Stayz

From the days when the developer of Airbnb couch-surfed at friend's places, Airbnb has grown into an worldwide empire that few would have imagined. Look on an Airbnb website and the accommodation can range from quirky to luxurious such as a camping spot, yurts, caravan, bus, yacht, granny flats, tree- houses to luxury houses.

So why do some people prefer Airbnb over hotels whilst others remain loyal to a particular hotel chain? Is it about saving money? Is Airbnb cheaper than hotels? Is it about staying in something a little unique and enjoying an experience as Airbnb is now promoting?

We have covered Airbnb as a business or additional source of income under the Finance chapter of this book so it may be helpful to revisit that chapter as we look further here.

When travelling, I like to mix my accommodation so that I will stay in some three-star hotels and, with the savings that I make there, I can then enjoy the luxury of a five or six-star hotel knowing that I am still within the overall budget set for the trip. I did this on a visit to San Francisco recently. I chose to stay a few nights on an Airbnb yacht near Pier 39 before having a couple of nights in a luxury hotel on Union Square.

So with any accommodation, and particularly when choosing Airbnb or a hotel, it is important to consider those you are travelling with, accommodation budget, where you are going and what you want to get out of the trip. In the example above, I wanted to be near the centre of San Francisco, close to transport and enjoy a few nights in a very upmarket hotel. I could not afford to stay the entire time in San Francisco at that hotel and so I looked for something cheaper. I looked at many options on Airbnb ranging from rooms to apartments and finally found the yacht. I liked the price (for San Francisco), I liked the location and it was something a little different – but it would not suit everyone.

Airbnb can allow you, given the right property, to cook some home-cooked meals. After a few weeks of eating in restaurants and other takeaways, a home-cooked meal is great. This also gives an opportunity to visit a local supermarket which can be a real eye-opener. On a trip to Berlin, I stayed in the old East Berlin area and went to a local supermarket. Labels on products were in German, Russian and Turkish but no English so there was a little pot luck as to what cans I chose. But it is all part of the travelling experience.

Hotels are excellent for short trips particularly for business when you may arrive late or depart early and housekeeping is available as are toiletries and 24-hour room service. Normally, they are well located for business as well as bars and restaurants if you have to do any entertaining. Hotels can also be useful when travelling with children with fold-out beds and children's meals available.

There is a common misconception that Airbnb is a cheaper source of accommodation. Price has been given as the number one consideration of why people book Airbnb. This is not necessarily correct so each proposed stay needs to be assessed on the nature of the trip. How many people are involved, the purpose of the trip, the accommodation requirements and your budget.

Research by Bank of America Morgan Stanley in 2015 suggests that using an Airbnb across the USA is a lot more expensive than a normal hotel. There are some exceptions in major cities like New York, Boston and Washington in the USA and overseas in cities like London, Berlin and Paris.

Airbnb has been promoted as the major disruptor to the hotel industry but it appears that the hotel industry has been able to adapt to the price changes brought about by Airbnb. The main areas that appear to be affected by Airbnb are the bed and breakfast, staying with family and friends and long-term stays in hotels.

It is important to understand any fees and charges that may be over and above the quoted fee for the period of the stay. There will also be an expectation of providing a review at the end of your stay as these might help the host achieve the sought-after title of Superhost.

Bed and Breakfasts (B&Bs)

As the name suggests, the traveller is given a bed and breakfast. B&Bs have been around in many countries for centuries but today they are threatened by the likes of Airbnb.

B&Bs are normally family homes or in some countries historic homes that are opened up to the public for a short stay, overnight or a couple of days. The owner of the property is generally the host and they provide the breakfast and other meals. They also undertake the cleaning. Normally a private room with a private bathroom is provided with breakfast being served in the bedroom, in the dining room or maybe on a verandah. Generally, there are only a small number of guests and it can provide a time to swap travel stories and places of interest to visit.

In most countries the B&Bs are regulated and some countries grade the establishments using a star rating issued by a national or state tourist organisation.

Hotels

The vast majority of hotel chains operate a loyalty program. These programs are normally based on the number of night stays as well as a revenue basis. The more nights and the more money spent in these hotels builds towards points and free nights. The more nights stayed also affects your status within the chain of hotels.

Your status may entitle you to a welcome drink, a free newspaper, free internet, late check-out or maybe a room upgrade or some combination.

As with airline status, it is important to consider the countries you may travel to, the style of the hotel accommodation you prefer and then join that hotel chain. Membership is generally free although there are some chains that have a membership fee. One chain in Australia charges in excess of $340 per year with the claim that you recoup this fee when you dine in their restaurants during the year.

Care needs to be taken when booking some of the cheaper hotels in the chains as they may not provide any benefits or status rewards.

Hotel breakfasts and car parking appear to be the cash cows for most hotel chains. Often, you will find a cheaper and more satisfying breakfast by taking a walk around to the nearby street.

Some hotels offer executive lounges and these often are value for money. If you have the required status, you will gain access to the executive lounge otherwise it is normally possible to book a room that gives you executive lounge access.

Many chains will, throughout the year, advertise special promotions for stays during certain periods for example, breakfast included in the room rate or breakfast for $1.

Sometimes there are also promotions to achieve a certain status level like gold. Instead of meeting the normal requirements to achieve the status level, the hotel may offer a fast track whereby you are required to stay a certain number of nights within a fixed timeframe such as 90 days. Depending upon the hotel chain, they may or may not allow you to enjoy the benefits of the status level that you are seeking to achieve.

Bed runs

As we have read with airline frequent flyer programs, there are some people that undertake status runs to obtain or keep their airline status level. There are also people with status with hotel loyalty programs that also undertake what is commonly called bed runs. They may not necessarily be travelling but, if they are short of a few nights, they may book into a hotel in the city in which they live for a weekend.

We have heard of more extreme situations where a person who holds highly valued elite status books into two hotels operated by the same hotel chain for the same night. It seems extreme, but some people highly value the status and benefits offered by the hotel.

Early morning flight arrivals

Because of Australia's geographical location, many of our overseas flights arrive in foreign countries late at night or early morning. Most hotels and Airbnb check-in times are after 2pm so what do you do if you have cleared customs and immigration by 5am?

If a traveller has status with an airline, they may be able to go to the arrivals lounge, have a shower and breakfast before heading towards their accommodation. Another alternative is to go to the hotel and drop off any luggage before going for a massage or sightseeing. Occasionally, if status is held with the hotel, early access may be given to your room. Airbnb is less likely to accommodate early arrivals. Another alternative is to pay for one extra night's accommodation so that you can access your room and catch up on some sleep.

Youth hostels

Many may remember staying in youth hostels around the world when they were a little younger. One that comes to mind immediately is a castle overlooking the Rhine River where my son, eleven years old at that time, would spend a few hours playing various card games with the other guests.

The good news is that youth hostels still exist and there is no upper age limit. The hostels provide bed, linen, blankets and cooking facilities but not a towel.

The level of accommodation will vary, depending upon the location, from a basic backpacker shared accommodation and facilities to family rooms.

Learning to pack

At the beginning, you need to remember that not all airlines will have the same baggage allowance so you need to pack for the one with the lowest allowance. Regardless of which country or airline you use, excess baggage charges are horrific.

We have had students stay with us for 3 – 6 months who bought things during that time and, despite what they were told, they had excess baggage when they departed. We know of a couple of students who had charges of around $800 and a friend of theirs had to leave one large suitcase behind because she could not afford the excess baggage charges.

If you are not sensible, excess baggage charges can cripple your travel budget. For most Australians, visiting the northern hemisphere during winter can be the most challenging as you need jumpers and overcoats, thermal underwear, thick socks, boots, scarves, beanies, gloves plus the essentials. At this point, the baggage allowance for an economy passenger is probably reached before any purchases of clothing, shoes or souvenirs overseas.

What is your style of packing? Some people pack as they go, perhaps over the course of a week or two and some others throw items onto the bed before packing them into the suitcase the night before departure. Some people fold as they pack and others roll? Which can you relate to?

Packing is an art form and needs to be learnt. Not only will inefficient packing cost you money, but haulage may also cause serious health problems such as muscle spasms, numbness in hands and arms and potential disc injuries. Anyone that has travelled around Europe will know how difficult the cobblestone streets and laneways can be when carrying or pulling luggage.

So how do you manage to pack correctly? As we have mentioned a few times in different chapters of this book, you need a plan or a strategy.

You need to know the worst-case scenario in terms of weight that will be allowed for each leg of the journey. Which airline, train, ferry or bus is going to have the most restrictions in terms of weight or number of bags allowed? This is then the maximum weight you need to work with unless you plan to leave some luggage with friends or in a storage locker for a short period. You need to be mindful of any low-cost airlines that you might use within a country as low-cost airlines typically have low baggage allowances. What can be taken on board as hand luggage and what is the weight allowed for hand luggage? What is the weight allowed for baggage that is to go into the hold of the aircraft? Also check with the airline website because some airlines have started to charge a fee for bags that are individually heavy. For example you may have an allowance of 28 kg but one bag may weigh 26 kg and the airline regards that as heavy and imposes a charge. If that luggage had been spread across 2 bags weighing 26 kg then there would be no charge.

The next step is to check the weather forecasts for each of the towns or cities you plan to visit. Having some idea of whether it is likely to rain or snow, whether the average temperature is in single figures or in the high 30's, and knowing the high and low forecast for each day will give some idea of what you need to pack. This can be challenging if embarking on a round the world trip but it is not impossible. For the round the world trips, you need to look at the number of days in each country to then get some idea of the proportions of clothing to pack.

Rather than fold and pack, it is a good idea to place all your clothing, shoes, books, toiletries, cameras and computer on a bed or on the floor over a few days or a week so that you get a good idea of what you propose to pack.

Think about how you may mix and match clothes to reduce the number of outfits required. If heading to colder weather, the idea is to layer the clothing worn so that you can reduce the number of heavy jumpers to be packed.

A good pair of comfortable walking shoes is essential if you are planning to do a lot of sightseeing and maybe another pair for going out to dinner. Do you need any more than that?

For males, a pair of jeans and maybe another pair of dark trousers that can be for both formal wear and casual when matched with a coat should suffice. I will not attempt to offer any advice for our female readers. If you can, plan out mix-and-match outfits for a week and then use the same outfits for the next week. If you are travelling around countries, the only person that will remember that you wore that outfit a week ago is you.

You also need to ask whether all the items on the bed or floor are needed and whether you have forgotten to include anything. Do you need a hair dryer, if staying in a hotel? Do you need both an iPad and a computer?

Prior to packing, consider the layout of the suitcase. Some suitcases with the retractable handle sliders divide into three rectangular areas and thus provide an opportunity to compartmentalise your clothing. Compartmentalisation makes it easier to find items and special packing cubes can also be useful for socks and underwear.

Rolling your clothes, rather than folding, will result in more items being packed. Socks and other small items can be placed inside shoes.

Even if leaving Australia in temperatures of 30 degrees and heading to the cold in the northern hemisphere, wear your heavy clothing and carry your overcoat onto the plane. This will help to reduce the weight of checked-in luggage and the overcoat will be useful when you arrive at your destination. Note also that some plane cabins can be chilly at certain times in the flight and some budget airlines do not provide blankets.

The next important thing to pack is cabin bags. Understand the rules of the airlines in regard to cabin bags. In Australia, both Qantas and Virgin are closely monitoring the weight and size of carry-on bags during the December and January period (at the time of writing). They are even using portable scales to check the bag weight of those passengers who bypassed the check-in counters by using online check-in and going straight to the boarding gate.

Because the luggage placed in the hold of the aircraft is possibly going through to your final destination, you might like to have a change of underwear and maybe more casual clothing in your carry-on bag. With toiletries, be mindful of the requirements for allowable sizes and having it placed in a clear plastic zip-lock bag. Having a change of underwear and some other clothes can also come in handy if one of your suitcases goes missing.

Today, we have all sorts of electronic gear that we must pack; mobile phone chargers, camera chargers, Kindle chargers, fast chargers, power bank battery and all the related cords. Try to keep these together and in a separate easily-identifiable soft container.

Your passport, airline tickets, itinerary, currency for your next destination, any medication required on the plane and pen should be readily accessible.

In case your passport, wallet or purse is stolen, it is a good idea to photocopy your passport, driver's licence and credit cards. Leave a copy at home with your next of kin and hide a copy in each of your bags. I also split any foreign currency that I have with my wife so that we have some if one of our wallets or purses is stolen.

Learn to travel in style for a fraction of the cost
The good news is that you can travel in style for just a fraction of the cost. We have shown you a number of ways to do that in the earlier pages.

There are a number of websites that provide information on travel, particularly regarding airlines. There are some online courses and at least one three-day workshop covering air travel and hotel accommodation. The courses appear to cost from a few hundred dollars for the online course to a few thousand dollars for the workshop.

It is said that one of the greatest experiences while travelling is tasting different local foods. To be able to taste the authentic foods, you will normally have to venture away from the tourist areas. Sometimes, you only have to go a few blocks away from the tourist strip to find the authentic restaurants and cafes frequented by the locals. If you don't feel like exploring, ask the hotel concierge. Otherwise be adventurous and walk around the streets. I did this in Rome and found a little restaurant filled with locals, a piano for entertainment and, even though English was not their first language, I managed to order a very delicious meal for a fraction of the cost of what I would have paid in my hotel or any of the restaurants nearby. If you can see the kitchen and it has older people cooking then you are also likely to get a great local meal. Generally, avoid restaurants with multi-language menus as you are probably still in tourist territory.

(Note: The author has status with airlines and hotels, has travelled extensively by train and visited over 30 countries to date so he has experienced being able to travel in style for a fraction of the cost).

Travel agents

Travel agents can provide a wealth of information on holiday destinations and bookings so they are very useful for most people when booking a holiday. They can provide some amazing deals and book some interesting accommodation. Travel agents traditionally received a commission on booking airfares, train, cruises, accommodation and car hire. Some travel agents now appear to be adding additional charges now so always check for any additional fees.

Over the years there have been a number of travel agencies that have closed their doors leaving holiday-makers thousands of dollars out of pocket. At the end of December 2018, another travel agency, Bestjet, an online budget travel agency, went into receivership leaving many customers without bookings or refunds. Their customers had paid the travel agent but the travel agent seemingly does not pay the airline until the passenger travels. The travel agent closed the doors, the airlines cancelled any bookings that they had not been paid for and the customers were left out of pocket with holiday plans in disarray.

More recently, we have had Thomas Cook in the United Kingdom close its doors.

Most travel insurance policies provide no cover for a travel agent going out of business and it appears that the International Air Transport Association (IATA) provides no protection either. If the customer uses a credit card to make the payment to the travel agent then they may have some success seeking a refund through a credit card chargeback. Some credit cards also provide travel insurance when airline fares are booked using the credit card.

What plans do you have for travel in retirement? Do you have a bucket list of destinations to visit? When do you plan to travel? Some people plan to do most of their travelling in the first five or seven years after retiring, while they are still fit and healthy.

The world is a large and interesting place. Start exploring but before you do, make sure you read the next chapter.

Key learnings from this chapter

Key learnings from this chapter

Chapter 10

Planning for the inevitable

Only two things are certain in life:death and taxes.

Benjamin Franklin

We spend precious hours fearing the inevitable. It would be wise to use that time adoring our families, cherishing our friends and living our lives.

Maya Angelou

Estate planning

This is simply a way of creating an orderly transfer of ownership and control of your assets in the event of your death or if an accident or illness was to leave you incapable of looking after your own affairs.

There may be secondary benefits to your beneficiaries in terms of reduced capital gains tax payable.

Estate planning has never been more important than it is today regardless of whether you have purchased rental properties, or invested in the share market. If you are buying, or own, a home or have superannuation, then you have an estate more valuable than maybe your parents and most certainly more than your grandparents. The second reason that estate planning is more important today is that in modern society blended families are very common.

Case study

Tom marries Mary and they have three children. Tom and Mary made a will shortly after they purchased a house but before any children had arrived. In their wills, they made each other beneficiaries of their respective estates. Tom dies unexpectedly and, in accordance with his will, Mary inherits his assets.

A few years later, Mary meets Jack and marries him. Jack has been divorced and has custody of his three children. After their marriage, Jack and Mary make new wills nominating each other as beneficiaries of their wills. Unfortunately Mary dies and Jack, as sole beneficiary, inherits Mary's estate. In the couple of years since Mary's death, Jack and his step-children are not getting on well together. One day when Jack realises that he no longer has a valid will, he makes a new will but leaves his estate to his (biological) children. Mary's children stand to inherit nothing. If Jack was to live for a long time and the rift between Jack and Mary's children remained unresolved, Jack could die and his will be uncontested by any of Mary's children. Alternatively, they could challenge the will and proceed with a costly legal contest.

You need to discuss rationally with your partner, preferably before marriage, how any assets owned are going to be distributed if either one should die. There are many combinations of how such a scenario with blended families could work. It depends on what assets are brought into the new marriage, who earns what, and whether there are any more children born into this blended family.

It is important to get this agreed to, preferably before marriage. Otherwise, it is likely that the only ones to win here will be solicitors because the children who feel they have missed out are likely to challenge the will.

Superannuation

We will not be going into detail about superannuation except to mention that superannuation does not form part of the estate covered by your will.

The trustees of your superannuation are responsible for distributing the funds in your superannuation account generally to the person you have nominated in your Binding Death Nomination but they do have some discretion.

Will

There seems to be reluctance by many people to have a will prepared. Maybe people are afraid of facing the reality of death or they feel that preparing a will may hasten the inevitable. Australia, over many years, has had a number of high-profile people like Robert Holmes a Court and Peter Brock die intestate; that is without a will. Dying intestate results in the estate being distributed according to the laws of the state or territory in which the deceased had lived. As was the case with Peter Brock's estate, this often leads to bitter legal battles where the only winners are the solicitors. Similarly, a low-cost 'Do It Yourself Will' may not provide the legally water-tight document that you desire and could be subject to a legal challenge. Wills being so important, I can never understand why solicitors do not provide a free will service for their clients at the time of undertaking conveyancing of a property. Instead they prefer to charge a few hundred dollars to create a will (as if they do not make enough out of the conveyancing).

What is a will and who are the main players?

Your will is a legal document that, upon your death, becomes a legally effective declaration of your wishes in terms of how you wish aspects of your estate to be handled. It may also cover such things as your burial or cremation and how your assets are to be distributed.

The requirements for a will are fairly simple. The person making the will should be at least 18 years old; although there are one or two exemptions. The person making the will should sign and date the document in the presence of two independent witnesses who must not be beneficiaries or a spouse of beneficiaries of the will. Correct witnessing of a will is essential otherwise it could become invalid if done incorrectly. The will must provide for the distribution of the whole of the estate. It can nominate specific items that you wish people to receive and it can be amended by attaching a document called a 'codicil'. The Oxford dictionary simply defines a codicil as an addition or supplement that explains, modifies or revokes a will or part of one.

Your will may be revoked:

1. by the creation of a new will
2. by intentionally destroying all copies of the document
3. by marriage or remarriage.

Note that divorce, by itself, does not change or cancel an existing will.

Your will can be prepared by a solicitor, by yourself using a Do It Yourself kit or by using the Public Trustee in some states and territories. The Public Trustee prepares the will free of charge but charges fees to administer the estate. Using a Public Trustee can be a costly alternative in the long term.

Because your will is the only legal document to convey your wishes after your death, it is important that it be drafted by a legally qualified person so that there is less likelihood of a dispute around the intention of words. A will can be rendered invalid by a small omission or an inconsistency. The goal of your will is to have your assets distributed to whomever you wish after your death.

The person or persons that you nominate to administer the will is known as your executor. Your executor has the responsibility of identifying all your assets and liabilities and then, in accordance with your instructions, distributing the net proceeds to the beneficiaries named in your will. In general, your executor has the final say over the administration of the will, unless it is challenged in court.

Surprisingly, wills and powers of attorney were not mentioned during all those years by the bank managers, financial planners and others that you may have come across in terms of monitoring your wealth. It is now common for financial planners to ask whether you have an up-to-date will. It is a topic of estate planning and one of the subjects covered in the Australian Diploma of Financial Planning.

If you were to die intestate, there is government legislation as to how your estate would be divided up with a certain percentage going to your wife and children. All bank accounts and other assets like property and shares that are in joint names, upon your death or the death of your spouse, would automatically transfer to the surviving partner.

Have you recently updated your wills and powers of attorney? It is important to have a say in how you wish your assets, assets that have taken a lifetime to accumulate, will be utilised after you have died rather than relying on the Government to distribute your estate. I believe that it is essential, and good stewardship, to have an up-to-date will clearly spelling out your wishes for your estate and which reflects your current situation.

It is important to revise and update your will whenever any significant changes happen in your family situation or wealth creation. Some significant changes that may result in a change in your will could include:

1. the birth or death of a child
2. the death of your spouse
3. marriage, divorce or bankruptcy
4. the purchase or sale of a business
5. a change in the beneficiary
6. an executor of your will dies, becomes incapacitated or bankrupt. (This is one reason why it is important to have a secondary executor).

In Australia and New Zealand, we are fortunate in that we do not have inheritance nor death duties whereby the Government takes a percentage of your wealth prior to distribution to your beneficiaries.

You can put as much or as little thought and time into your will as you wish. A very simple will may leave everything to your spouse and/ or to your surviving children.

But things can get complicated for a number of reasons. For example, with blended families, if there is a situation with substance abuse by a potential beneficiary and whether there are any grandchildren, or the likelihood of grandchildren, to name a few.

It is important to get legal advice in establishing your will so that your assets are distributed in accordance with your wishes. Equally important, but harder to do, is to have a family conference to explain to your spouse and children the broad details and the rationale of your will.

If you wish to leave your assets to your children and grandchildren, your solicitor may suggest a testamentary trust. A testamentary trust manages assets in your will after your death, distributing both income and capital according to your instructions. Testamentary trusts can result in tax savings to beneficiaries; maintaining social security payments to the surviving spouse and income splitting to younger children. It may also protect assets if a beneficiary is declared bankrupt. The disadvantage of testamentary trusts is that it adds a further degree of complexity to the will and it is only as good as current legislation so a change to government legislation in the future could diminish the current benefits.

Apart from covering how your financial affairs are to be distributed to your spouse, children, grandchildren, or bequests and gifts to charities, you can attach a letter to your will to cover your wishes in terms of donating organs and/or tissue. The instructions or directions that are contained in this letter are not binding; it is only an expression of your wishes. It is best to have had a discussion with your immediate family beforehand so that it is clear what your wishes were in this regard.

A will can eliminate a lot of stress and wasted money if your wishes are clearly known.

Do not forget to review your will regularly in case you want to change beneficiaries, or bequests, as your estate changes.

Assets not included in your will

We have already mentioned that your superannuation is not covered by your will. If you have used a family trust in which to own shares or property, these are also not owned in your name and therefore not covered by your will. Also assets owned in joint names automatically transfer to the surviving owner. Assets owned by a private company are not included in the will but the shares in the company owned by the deceased can be left in the will.

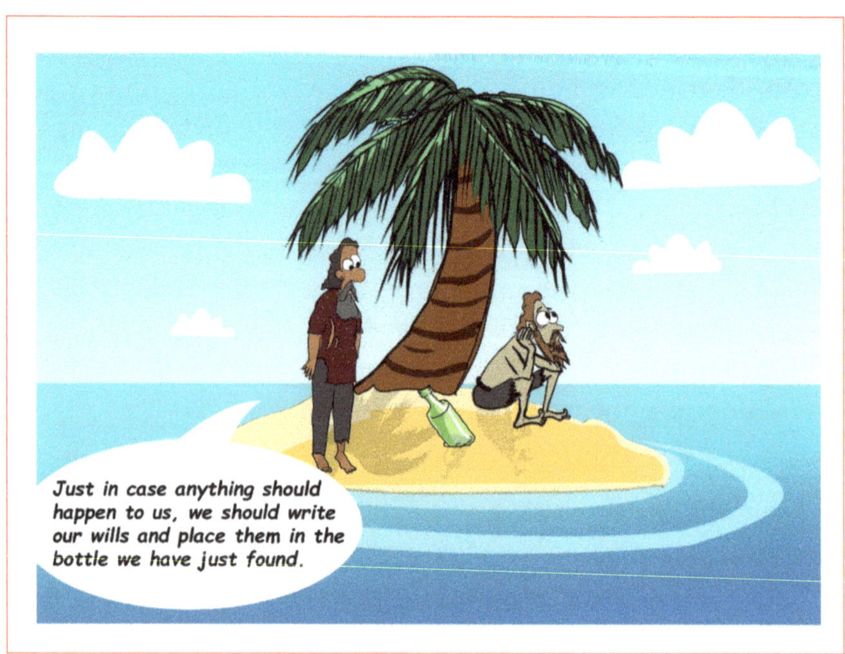

Power of attorney

This is basically a written authority giving another person or persons the authority to act on your behalf and to conduct your affairs. The authority can be for a limited period or activity. For example, while travelling overseas, you may give a person a power of attorney to act on your behalf if you are in the process of selling a property in Australia. You can decide whether the power of attorney you give is to be wide or narrow in scope and for how long it is to run; for example, only while travelling overseas for six weeks. A power of attorney can also be for a long period of time once a certain condition occurs. For example, if there is an accident or illness that results in the person not being capable of managing their affairs, then the holder of the power of attorney can make decisions on behalf of that person including the buying and selling of property, paying bills, filing tax returns and directing investments.

You can revoke a power of attorney at any time provided you are still of sound mind. Your ordinary power of attorney remains valid only while you are alive and still mentally capable.

It is important that the person/s you choose to be your power of attorney is/are totally trustworthy. You can have different powers of attorney for different areas; for example, one for financial affairs and another for health-related matters.

Note:

Preparing for the inevitable by having a will and power of attorney prepared and also working on your legacy does not mean you are giving up on life. Far from it. But they are prudent steps if you want to retain some control at a time when you are not physically capable.

Advance Health Directive

Advanced Health Directive (AHD) is a document that contains your wishes about your future health care for various medical conditions and comes into effect only if you are unable to make your own decisions regarding health care. An AHD made in one state or territory is valid in other states and territories although there may be some differences in treatment. Each state or territory has slightly different requirements for the AHD so it is recommended that you check the requirements in the state in which you live or in which you plan to live.

AHDs are made by people who feel it is important to specify what treatments they want, or do not want, in the future based on religious beliefs, past experience with a loved one or from talking with other people or medical professionals.

An AHD can be made by anyone over the age of 18 with the legal capacity to understand the nature and effect of the health directive. At the time of making the directive, the person's decision-making must not be affected by alcohol, drugs, medication nor impaired by illness, disease or injury. The AHD must be made by the person for whom it is intended, not by another person under instruction.

Once made, the AHD remains in force until revoked or changed. It is recommended that the AHD be reviewed every two years or if the person's health changes significantly. To change an AHD, a new form can be completed and the old form destroyed. To revoke an AHD, no formal form is required; just written instructions revoking the AHD. These written instructions are to be witnessed.

Because of the complex nature of the decisions being made about health treatment, it is recommended that you make an appointment with a doctor to go through the various options regarding future treatment so that you understand everything. Other doctors, at the time of providing treatment based on the AHD, will feel more confident to follow the directive knowing that decisions have been made in consultation with a doctor.

If you do not have an AHD, medical staff will always work to prolong life. If illness or accident results in an irreversible condition or persistent vegetative state, then doctors will consult your next of kin with recommendations that they feel are best for all concerned.

Simplify life

Being an executor of a will can be a difficult role. You can simplify life for the executor by closing unused or little used bank accounts and credit cards that are no longer required and putting all important documents together in a box or a filing cabinet.

Pets are an important part of our lives, particularly as we age, so it is important to think about who may look after your pets when you are gone.

Talk to your family also about who is prepared to look after you if you have treatment for, say, cancer. If you have a choice of where you would like to die, would you prefer to be at home, in a hospice or in a hospital?

Talking things through with your family is important and you may need to have the conversation more than once.

Donating organs

In Australia, you have a fantastic opportunity to help and save other people after you have died. You can donate your heart, lungs, liver, kidneys and pancreas as well as tissues such as corneas, heart valves, bone and skin to be used in life-saving operations.

Have no fear, a doctor's first priority is to save lives and, unless you have given instructions not to be resuscitated, then the medical staff will work tirelessly to save your life. They will not be switching off your life support prematurely. You can be comforted to know that the doctors will, in fact, perform more tests than usual to confirm that you really are dead before harvesting any organs.

It is vitally important that your family knows your wishes in regard to organ donations because, even if you are on the organ donation register, your family can override your wishes if they are uncertain.

You should never assume that you are too old or unfit to be a donor. Be registered as a donor (there is a National Donor Register) and allow doctors to make decisions as to what organs they may be able to use.

If you are into recycling while you are alive, what better recycling example to set your family than to donate your organs or your body?

Donating your body

Sometimes this is referred to as 'leaving your body to science'. Bodies are used by universities to teach a number of disciplines about the human body, not just doctors and dentists. There are very strict guidelines as to how donated bodies are used and, at the end of a specified period (normally 2–4 years), your body is cremated or buried in a public burial ground not accessible to the public for visitations. But there are a number of things to consider and it is best to have a contingency plan…..

If you are considering leaving your body to science, you should contact a university that has medical teaching facilities. The university will provide a donor form to be completed and this should be done in consultation with the immediate family so that they are aware of your wishes. Once the university has processed the donor form, they will send confirmation and a donor card. It should be noted that an entry in your will to donate your body to science is too late to be acted upon and universities require your approval on the donor form. Generally, if any member of your family objects to your body being donated, then the university will not accept your body regardless of your will or donor form.

Even though the university has approved you as a donor, it does not mean that your body will be accepted. If the university has sufficient bodies for their needs then they will not accept any more. Your death also needs to occur within a designated area close to the university and someone will need to notify the university immediately of the death so that your body can reach the university in a timely manner; normally within 24 hours and no more than 48 hours after death. Each university has their own rules governing body donations…..

If your death was due to a significant disease then your body will not be accepted. Once your remains reach the university, a range of tests for diseases such as hepatitis, HIV, mad cow disease and tuberculosis, as well as about two dozen other diseases, will be undertaken. If a positive result occurs for any of these diseases, your body will be rejected.

The universities will also not accept your body if it has been used for donating body parts or an autopsy has been performed as they require complete bodies.

Some tissues and body parts may be kept indefinitely by the university. The remainder of the body is kept until the university has finished with the remains and then they are disposed of, as noted before, at the university's expense.

For the family, a memorial service, minus coffin, can be held to provide some closure. However, for some family members, closure may not occur for 2–4 years until the university has finished with the remains and burial or cremation has occurred.

It is a major decision to donate your body to science. It requires many people to know your wishes, for those wishes to be carried out without delay after your death, and for you to have no diseases that would exclude your body from being accepted.

Funeral service

Do you have any ideas of how you would like your funeral service to be conducted – if you want one at all? Have you spoken to your family about it? Often, this is not a subject that is raised and, if it is raised, other members of the family are likely to say that you are far too young to be thinking about such things.

It is, however, something that you may want to think about even if it is just to save your family some stress at the time of your death. They are likely to have enough things to think about: family and friends to contact, which funeral home to contact, what type of coffin or casket, where the service is to be held, burial or cremation, who may conduct the service, where to hold a wake, etc.

You may want to think about some of these things and write them down. It does not have to be done in a day; you can think about it over a period of time and make amendments as things become a little clearer over time.

You can possibly look for a venue for a service or the wake; pick the music, favourite songs, a poem or a passage from a favourite book. You can think about whom you would like to deliver the eulogy and maybe even write your own eulogy. With video facilities available on mobile phones, consider recording a farewell message that could be played at your funeral service. Do you have favourite clothes that you would like to be buried or cremated in?

Funeral costs

Funerals are becoming big business with just a few large companies controlling much of the funeral business in Australia. These large companies have been buying out the small family businesses that had traditionally run funeral homes so today there is very little competition.

It is hard not to notice advertising on radio and television for prepaid funerals, starting from as little as a few dollars per week, to give your loved ones peace of mind.

These policies are not new. One of my grandfathers took out a policy shortly after arriving in Australia, paying in regular amounts, and when he died some 15 years later, the estate received a relatively small amount towards the funeral costs.

Having experienced first-hand, a number of times, an unexpected death and organising a funeral, I can say from experience that it is not easy to decide on such things as a casket or coffin, funeral or cremation, flowers, funeral notices, etc. Even a very simple funeral costs money so the idea of having funds available to pay for your funeral is a valid one. The question is then whether it is best to join a funeral fund to prepay your funeral or to put money aside in a bank account administered by yourself and your future executors.

If you are looking at an Australian pension as part of your retirement planning then it is important to look at this question as there are rules around what can be paid for and how.

Burial, cremation or other

What happens with your body is sometimes based on cultural or religious beliefs and, at other times, based on personal preference. Many thousands of years ago, the Neanderthals started burying their dead in the ground, the Egyptians used sarcophagi, Ancient Greeks used clay urns, and the Romans carved coffins out of limestone. In India, cremation occurs on the banks of the Ganges.

In Australia, there are a number of options such as burial, cremation and burial at sea as well as giving your body to science. No longer is it just a wood coffin or casket; we now have cardboard coffins made from recycled paper and non-toxic chemicals. In some places, headstones are being replaced by trees.

If planning a sea burial, be prepared to work through red tape.

For those concerned about the planet and thinking about cremation, there are several considerations…..

It takes about 2-3 hours to cremate an average body so consider the power used to achieve this. Much of the mercury in the atmosphere comes from burning amalgam fillings in teeth. If the body has been embalmed, which is common in many countries, and then the body is cremated, what happens to the embalming fluids like highly toxic formaldehyde, glutaraldehyde and methanol?

Leaving a legacy

When speaking of a legacy, most people will think of money and say that they have nothing to leave future generations.

A legacy to future generations does not need to involve money. In fact, a non-financial legacy may be more important than any monetary legacy that you could leave…..

For those with computer skills, consider setting up a personal web page, writing blogs and podcasts for your family. This provides a permanent time capsule for future generations.

For others who are able to leave a financial legacy, what would you do? In Queensland, a nurse,who died in 2017, left a third of his estate to be divided among the mourners who attended his funeral. His executors had the task of finding approximately 200 people who attended his funeral, providing his last surprise to them and thanking them for their friendship!

The Baby Boomers as children

A large number of the Baby Boomers had grandparents who were in their early to mid-fifties when their grandchildren were being born. This gave the grandchild and grandparents a number of years to bond, to get to know each other and spend time together. Many were immigrants from Britain or Europe who, having been through the depression and then the world war, came to Australia to make a new start and provide a better life for their children.

The grandparents of the Baby Boomers were generally not wealthy, having modest homes, a Holden, Falcon or Chrysler car and some savings. Retirement was at age 65 for males and 60 for females and, with no superannuation, the government pension was generally their sole source of income. Whole of Life insurance policies were popular investments and I can remember one of my grandfathers reaching the age of 80 and receiving a cheque paying out his Whole of Life insurance policy. I can't remember the amount that he received but it was not a large sum of money for the length of time that he had been paying into the policy; but my grandfather was happy that he had lived long enough to get some money back from the insurance company.

While they did not have a great deal of money, the grandparents of the Baby Boomers generally had the precious commodity of time available to spend with their grandchildren. I well remember one of my grandfathers teaching me how to tell the time using the wall clock.

The children of the Baby Boomers are getting married and having children later in life so, for many of us, we may be in our sixties before any grandchildren arrive. Unless we have great genes, there is no chance of meeting any great-grandchildren.

Why not also write a letter to your spouse, to your sons and your daughters or grandchildren? There is no right or wrong way to do this. You can write whatever you feel like.

I started writing to my grandchildren long before any grandchildren arrived. I have told them a little about me, their grandmother, their father and mother, aunts and uncles and the lives that we live. Even if I am lucky enough to meet them, I don't know if they will be old enough to remember me so it is my way of letting them know a little about me, our family and my wishes for them as they grow.

Start recording your memories while they are still vivid. You can write them down, make audio recordings, maybe a video or a combination of these.

The letters to your spouse, sons and daughters can again be anything that you would like them to remember – reminiscence of the good times, wishing them well and providing some encouragement for the future and how proud you are of their achievements to date.

Hopefully you have some ideas now and want to put pen to paper or start a Word document. Your letter does not necessarily have to be written at one time – start now and add to it later as the years go by.

For those who are financially able, is there any particular cause that may be considered? Could you manage a bequeath to the Salvation Army, Lifeline, or establish a scholarship? I have heard of people building a school, or buying a goat or cow for a village in under-developed countries that they had visited during their lifetime. You do not need to have millions of dollars or the wing of your local hospital named after you to be able to provide a legacy.

Key learnings from this chapter

Key learnings from this chapter

Chapter 11

What does your retirement plan look like?

We work all our lives so we can retire – so we can do what we want with our time – and the way we define or spend our time defines who we are and what we value.

Bruce Linton

There is a fountain of youth: it is your mind, your talents, the creativity you bring to your life and the lives of people you love. When you learn to tap this source, you will truly have defeated age.

Sophia Loren

So far we have looked at the financial aspects of retiring, the psychology and health, ways of reinventing yourself, where you might live, travel, and preparing for the inevitable. Now it is time to pull it all together into your retirement plan. Talking with those that are now retired, the consensus is that those who had planned their transition from employment to retirement had a more satisfying life than those who had no plan. Pre-retirees and retirees were more confident, happier and successful in retirement when they had a detailed retirement plan.

Before starting, think about:

1. Your beliefs and goals
2. What do you truly believe in?
3. Are there any causes that you are passionate about – ending poverty, child slavery, saving the planet or volunteering at your local charity?

4. What can you do to further these causes?
5. What do you really want out of your life?
6. What legacy do you want to leave?

By now, you should have an idea of a retirement date, or at least know the year, and therefore know how many years or months you have before that day arrives. You will also have a far better idea of how much money you will need in retirement and what your starting base is. You are therefore well ahead of most Australian retirees who arrive at retirement with little knowledge or thought about their finances, health or housing.

We have found that, for the planning sessions, it is good to get away somewhere, away from the domestic distractions, the possibility of family and friends dropping in unannounced. Is there a favourite park or beach where you can sit, contemplate and write?

To get through the work required, it is good to have an agenda and a timetable as there is a lot to cover; health, relationships, travel, accommodation and leisure. To start with, think about where you see yourself in 10 years' time at a fairly broad level and then become more descriptive at 5 years, 3 years and 1 year – and very detailed at 90 days. This is the action plan to start moving towards your 10-year vision; the process is about strategic thinking not problem solving.

We have all planned for things throughout our lives such as significant birthdays, weddings, holidays or buying a house or car. Planning is simply a process of getting from A to B, whether a trip or an event; you are moving from an idea to the event happening.

Any planning process normally can be categorised into four main stages:

1. Pre-planning
2. Commitment

3. Implementation
4. Reviews

The chapters leading up to this point have detailed the pre-planning that needs to be considered in planning for our retirement. If you feel unsure about a certain area, it is worth revisiting that chapter.

Pre-planning

Each person will have a different focus on the pre-planning depending upon:

1. their stage in life,
2. their wealth status and
3. what they want in retirement.

Remember, wealth is more than just financial. Your wealth also includes your health, relationships and your ability to enjoy your life. There is no right or wrong in developing the retirement plan. It is what you and your partner want and feel comfortable with. Not everyone has a desire to travel or a desire to be a millionaire owning multiple properties or a large share portfolio. For many, this would be replacing the shackles of a job with the shackles of constantly monitoring a portfolio of shares or property. Some do not see a great future in retirement. We hope that this book has dispelled many of those thoughts. You may now feel that there is a great deal to do in retirement and have set a goal to live to 100 and receive the telegram from our head of state, whoever that may be in the future.

Remember, in retirement you need a reason to get out of bed each morning so what will inspire you to do that? What will push your boundaries and help you make a difference in the world?

There is a concept in psychology called 'self-continuity' whereby you imagine yourself in the future. It appears that it dates back to the ancient Greeks and scientists who believed that you are better off if you can connect to this future self. Think about the following questions under each of the different age brackets:

Self Continuity questions examples				
Question	60–70 years	70–80 years	80–90 years	Over 90 years
How is my relationship with my partner?				
What exercises should I do?				
What travel will I do?				
Where do I live?				
Remaining space for your questions for your life				

So what type of retirement do you envisage for yourself? Are you going to be fit and healthy with a good circle of friends and family, financially free, living where you want to live and the lifestyle that you want? What is on your bucket list? Have you identified and prioritised the things you want for your life? Do you have any major plans or projects like house renovations or an extended holiday overseas?

Have you created a bucket list of things to see and do? What is on your bucket list;

1. cruise around the world?
2. fly in a helicopter or a glider?
3. go on a safari in Africa?
4. a trip on the Orient Express?

5. work on the family tree?
6. learn to play a musical instrument? and
7. learn to paint or make pottery?
8. learn yoga or tai chi?
9. volunteer work each week? or
10. spend more time with the grandchildren?

Not everything has to cost money to be on your bucket list.

I recently read about another list called a 'curious list' which is a list of things that you are interested in and may like to consider learning at some time in retirement. For example, you may have had a long interest in flying and a desire to learn to fly but now your age or health would prevent you from obtaining your pilot's licence. If it was on your curious list, you could still explore how planes fly, obtain all the details of what pilots must learn to pass their pilots licence and even spend some time in a flight simulator. Without spending thousands of dollars to obtain your pilot's licence, you now understand all that is required to fly a plane.

Let's look at your current financial position:

1. What do you own and what do you owe?

2. What is your income and what do you spend?

3. Do you need to focus or have a plan to eliminate any debt like credit cards or mortgage?

4. Do you need to reassess what you spend?

5. Do you have any major plans like a house renovation or plans for an extended holiday?

Are there things that you are currently doing which may use current resources such as time or money that are not providing any long-term benefit towards your goals? Whether they are big or small items, if they are not part of your retirement plan then consider stopping that activity.

At this stage, let's summarise some goals for each area of your life:

Area of life:				Date:
Goal	Next 12 months	1–5 years	5-10 years	10 years plus

Consider creating a vision board to illustrate your future. A vision board is simply a collage of images and words that have meaning to you and which inspire and motivate you.

Another way to approach the visualisation of your retirement is to write a letter to your future self. You can describe your life now and then think about the type of person you are and what you want to say to your future person in 10-15 years' time.

These goals help to define the path you wish to follow now and in the future. What you want to do will impact you financially; your health and finances may also significantly impact on your goals. Creating your dream retirement requires an achievable plan. Try to imagine what a week, month, year or decade may look like in your retirement. It is important that your expectations of retirement are not too high or too low as both can lead to demotivation in retirement and influence how you adapt in retirement.

Committing to a plan

Experts tell us that any goals have to be written down and in ink, not pencil. The same principle applies to a plan. Writing your plans helps to clarify your ideas. Having it in ink refers to a permanency and stability in that it is not as easy to change. Look at the goals that you have written down.

Have you considered factors that may be beyond your control?

1. Losing your job
2. Serious long term illness and how these events may affect your plans.
3. If you are planning to sell some property or shares, how does <u>not</u> selling within the timeframe or within the set price range affect your plans? Remember, there is market risk and market cycles to consider. What are your contingencies?

The format of your written plan is up to you. Some people may write it as a letter to themselves, some may write it as if these things have already happened and others may list action items under headings. Again, there is no right or wrong – it is what you are comfortable with and are likely to achieve.

The plan should have your starting point, where you are today and what you want to achieve, a timeframe and steps to achieving this. You may have a master plan and individual plans for the various areas of your life as you focus on health, friends and family, finances, travel and housing. Do you have a long-term strategy for achieving your plan and the things on your bucket list? Have you broken down the master plan for each area of your life into manageable and measurable areas? Do you need to assess your resources such as finances and time both now and into the future? The resources available, and used, will be different for various stages leading up to, and into, retirement.

Set a date for reviewing your plans to ensure you are on target or make any necessary adjustments for things in your life that may have changed. Take time to think about how possible scenarios may impact on your various plans, what could be a worst case scenario and what compromises or changes may need to be made. In chapter 1, we saw that 33 per cent of men and 20 per cent of women had little or no control over when they retired due to illness, disability or retrenchment. What is your plan B that covers for such unforeseen happenings?

What are the risks associated with doing, or not doing, various parts of the plan? For example, with exercise there is the risk of injury if not undertaken properly but the penalty for not exercising is that there is an increased risk of heart and other chronic diseases.

In the preface we mentioned that:

1. Only about 62 per cent of survey respondents had some kind of financial plan,
2. 24-27 per cent had some plans for health and
3. 17-26 per cent had plans for their lifestyle, social and community engagement.

Preparing your plans will place you well ahead of most pre-retirees and ready to enjoy the benefits of your retirement.

Implementation

Planning your dream retirement is important but it will only remain a dream unless you combine knowledge and action to make it a reality. This is your life and your plan to implement therefore we are only going to provide some prompts under the various headings for you to think about as you write your plan. Remember, you can have all the greatest goals and ideas in the world but unless they are implemented, they remain just goals and ideas.

While you may not want to admit it, some of the things that you miss the most in retirement will be the structure, purpose and direction given by employment. You need to set schedules and routines in retirement to replace them. What type of schedules and routines might you have?

Financial

Having identified your retirement lifestyle and allocated a dollar figure, now is the time to develop a portfolio to achieve it.

1. Take a long-term view of your investments
2. Critically examine each investment.
3. Does the investment provide long-term income, capital growth or both?
4. Do you have investments that are defensive, income or growth assets?
5. Develop a diversified portfolio as this will decrease risk over the longer term.
6. Remember, even the safest investment vehicle must achieve one basic objective – beating inflation.

A common mistake by retirees is to completely change their investment mix once they retire to focus on income generation. Rather than have major changes, it is best to have a consistent approach to your investment mix prior to, and in, retirement. This will help smooth out short-term fluctuations. Changes in your portfolio, whether buying or selling, will cost money.

Review your current assets and expenditure:

1. Are there any shares or property that you need to sell either because of poor performance or limited capital growth?
2. Do you need to consider selling some assets to pay down debt leading into retirement?
3. If you have two cars, do you need both? How much can you save in registration and insurance by selling one car?
4. Consider reducing the number of credit cards you have
5. What purchases are made on the credit card?
6. Are they paid off monthly? Get into the habit of paying off the credit card balance each month so that you are not paying any interest on these purchases.
7. Consider whether memberships are worth continuing. Often you will have small monthly charges going onto your credit cards for services that you no longer need.

Now is the time to review your insurances – life, income protection, disability insurance, trauma insurance, car, boat, caravan, house, content and health.

1. Do you need the insurance for example income protection or disability insurance? or
2. The level of insurance that you have? If the mortgage is now paid off or significantly reduced, do you need the insurance cover that you took out when you were in debt?
3. Do you know what your insurance is costing you each year?
4. When was the last time you compared companies and coverage?

Have you consolidated all your superannuation into one account? Consolidation is likely to save on fees. Have you compared the performance and fees charged of your superannuation fund with other funds? Do you need to change superannuation funds?

There may also be some new expenditure like gym membership so factor any new expenditure associated with your new life as a retiree into your budget.

Will you be entitled to a pension or part-pension? Do you qualify for any concessions? When will you be able to access these?

Health

Numerous surveys have shown that health is the number one priority for retirees – higher than overseas travel. Have a health check to establish your baseline then work on your physical, mental health and dietary requirements. Exercises like walking, golf, bowls and swimming are good but also think about core strength, balance, etc. Establish a weekly exercise routine.

To recap on areas that we covered in the chapter on health:

1. Do you have a plan for annual health and dental checks?
2. Have you had scans for bone mineral density and heart?

3. Have you had a colonoscopy?
4. Do you have a family history of health issues that need to be checked, for example high blood pressure or diabetes?
5. Do you exercise?
6. How often and with whom? Exercising with a partner will be more enjoyable and hold you accountable to do the exercise.
7. What mental stimulation do you undertake to keep the brain active?
8. Do you need to change the food that you eat, the amount that you eat or drink that you consume?
9. Are you eating five serves of vegetables and two serves of fruit a day?
10. Are you drinking sufficient water?

Friends and relationships

Friends and relationships will change over time. Unfortunately, as part of life, you will lose friends as they move away or pass away. You may also be blessed with new family members such as grandchildren. You must also work on your relationship with your spouse, your children and grandchildren.

Unfortunately, statistics suggest that your children's marriages may end in divorce so be mindful of the possibility.

Friendships are important:

1. Do you have a plan to make new friends?
2. Are you developing your own friends separately from those of your partner?
3. How do you meet new people?
4. Have you contacted old friends, including those from school days?

It may take time but good relationships are important.

Housing

What is important now, and as you get older, may change.

Have you considered;

1. The importance of public transport and closeness to shops and cinemas ?
2. Do you want to be closer to your children and grandchildren?
3. Is the house too big for you?
4. The cost of selling such as agent fees, removal costs and the buying costs of stamp duty, legal fees etc.?
5. A retirement village or similar and do you and your family fully understand the upfront and ongoing costs?
6. What renovations or modifications might need to be undertaken in the near future to allow you to remain in the home?
7. A reverse mortgage may provide capital in retirement but make sure that your children are aware of your intention and fully discuss the implications with an independent accountant.
8. Overseas students living with you? They provide company, they can be mentally stimulating and provide some income.
9. Airbnb as a source of additional income?

Travel

It is easy to think of the travel that you might do in the first year of retirement but remember you are likely to have twenty or more good years to travel.

When considering travel, have you:

1. Got a bucket list of places to visit whether Australia, New Zealand or overseas? As you talk to other people, there may be countries that you have not considered visiting but you can always research and add them to your list.
2. Prioritised travel to certain destinations as some areas that you plan to travel to may be more physically challenging therefore you should plan to visit these countries earlier.

3. Set a goal of taking your grandchildren on their first overseas trip, maybe back to their ancestral homeland? At what age would you do that and how many years is that away?
4. Researched and joined the frequent flyer program for the airline or airline alliance that you are likely to travel with?
5. Researched and joined the hotel program/s that will meet your travel needs both in Australia and overseas?
6. Researched and joined the loyalty programs for any cruise or tour companies?
7. Undertaken any study of airlines and hotels to understand how to gain status, buy points or miles in order to reduce your travel costs?

Wills and power of attorney

A brief recap on this important topic.

Do you?

1. Have a current will and power of attorney?
2. Stay in contact with your executors and are they all still alive?
3. Have a replacement executor, if you should require one?
4. Do you have an advance health directive?
5. Need to update your will if there have been any major changes to your assets or marital status ?

Remember your superannuation is not covered by your will so ensure that you have a current binding nomination. Binding nominations need to be updated every three years.

Any family trusts or other trusts are also not covered in your will.

Review

Change is inevitable and constant; your life will change hopefully for the better but there will always be hiccups along the way. So it is important that you set time aside to review your plan regularly. You may decide to do this every six months, or annually, so develop a habit and make a diary note to do it. People make New Year resolutions on New Year's Eve so in the lead-up, or in the days just after, is this a time of year to do your review?

Apart from an annual review, it may also be worth looking at your plan when the federal and state budgets are handed down to see if these budgets have any implications for your plan, particularly your financial plan. Your financial plan may be the simplest to review.

Things to consider when reviewing your plans:

1. Are you achieving the desired outcomes?
2. Any changes in your risk profile?
3. How changes in your other plans may affect your financial plans.
4. Do you need to change your asset allocation if there is a downturn in shares or property or, if one of those areas has boomed?
5. Do you feel you have disproportionate holdings in one sector or the other?

It is always good looking back on a plan to see what has been accomplished and what is still to be achieved. Are there new goals that you have set that need to be updated in your plans?

The plan is <u>your</u> plan so make changes to it as required. You can delete things that no longer hold any further appeal and add new adventures. Who would have thought that man landing on the moon would open up the possibility of tourism to the moon? Some people would love to go to the moon and are healthy and have the financial resources to be able to afford the cost for a return trip. Are you one of those people?

Has staying fit now encouraged a new goal of competing in the masters' games?

Continue to develop new relationships and monitor for loneliness and depression.

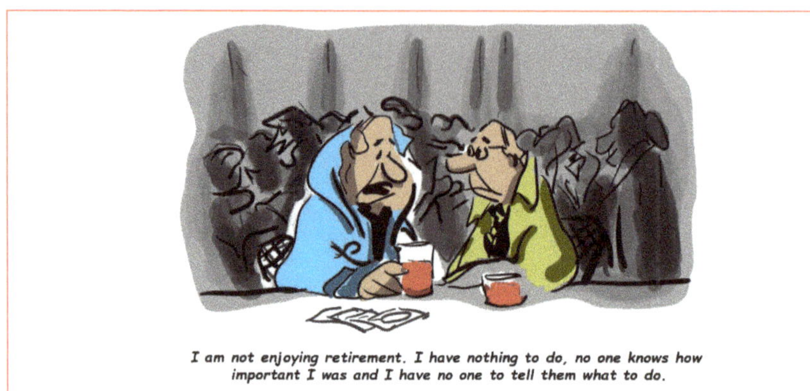

Closing thoughts

Retirement, as your parents and grandparents knew it, is dead. You are entering new frontiers, the unknown. Never before has such a large part of the population been faced with such a dilemma as what your retirement is going to look like.

Your parents and grandparents generally had a relatively short retirement during which time they may have had some travel and spent time with their grandchildren before moving to an aged person's home and dying. The pension was adequate for their lifestyle particularly as life expectancy was relatively short and the family home, their main asset, provided a small legacy for the children.

Today, you no longer have to retire at a set age if you want to keep working. If you do decide to retire then you need to finance your retirement for at least 20-30 years. You also need to remain healthy so that you can enjoy those years.

Preparation is the cornerstone to a happy and fulfilling retirement. We need to prepare emotionally, physically, psychologically as well as financially. We need a positive mental attitude, an ability to handle change and a determination to get on with the rest of our lives.

Retirement can be whatever you want it to be. It can be a time to relax, travel and endless leisure pursuits or to try something new and challenging. It's your life – go and enjoy it.

Chapter 12

Coronavirus (Covid19)

Expect the unexpected. Nobody saw Covid19 coming, nor what effect it would have worldwide.

Some words and phrases like unprecedented, new normal, stimulus, 'in this together' have become commonplace over the last 12 months. Many of us have learnt a little history regarding the Spanish flu and quarantine stations in Australia.

We had planned to have a launch for this book on 15 April 2020 but, like so many other events that had to be cancelled due to Covid19, our book launch was also cancelled. With our printers in Melbourne, our book was unable to be printed during the lockdowns.

Since then, I have been approached to write an additional chapter for the book, specifically on Covid19 and how this has affected areas that we have mentioned in the book. Writing this chapter has taken 12 months; it has been written and rewritten many times as Covid19 keeps affecting our lives. Like many things in our lives, it has brought out the good and bad in people. We look overseas at the terrible effects and death toll that Covid19 has had, we rejoice in how well Australia and New Zealand have coped but then we have an outbreak resulting in lockdowns and we want to turn on our politicians for trying to keep us safe. Yes, there have been some individuals that have done the wrong things but, overall, Australians have banded together to keep Covid19 reasonably well under control. Eradication is unlikely.

Covid19 is likely to be with us for a long time yet, although some vaccines are now available overseas and will be in Australia from about March 2021. We still don't know what the side effects, if any, of these vaccines may be or how often they may be required or what the long term effects of Covid19 might be. So, after 12 months of living with Covid19, what can we learn and how can it be applied to our planning for retirement?

Despite your political views, it has to be acknowledged that Australia has done exceptionally well in handling the health issues of the pandemic. Australia, compared with other countries, has also come through reasonably well economically. Yes, like the rest of the world, Australia will have a massive debt to deal with over the coming years or decades; our unemployment has almost tripled but is now falling faster than many predicted. Australia joined other countries and entered into a recession, the worst since the Great Depression of the 1930s. In many ways, we are in uncharted waters. We are not just dealing with an economic issue like we experienced in 2007-09 with the Global Financial Crisis; we are also dealing with a pandemic.

It was an interesting approach that the Morrison Government took to addressing Covid19 – establishing Team Australia comprising the Prime Minister, the Premiers of each State and the Chief Ministers of each Territory. Unfortunately, what started out as a united front to the pandemic started to unravel after just a few months. States and territories closed their borders, Victoria, and in particular Melbourne, had a second outbreak which belatedly resulted in a prolonged shutdown and, all the while, the Federal Government and New South Wales were calling for the borders to reopen. All our leaders, whether state or Commonwealth, followed the advice of health professionals - unlike some overseas countries.

Some 50 countries like Australia launched digital contract tracing apps although the one in Australia seems to have been far from successful in tracing where people had been if they were found to have the virus.

In early 2020 the Australian Government quickly identified the virus as a potential pandemic. One can only speculate how

Australia would have fared if the passengers from the Ruby Princess had been stopped from disembarking or if the Australian Government had waited until the World Health Organisation had declared a pandemic.

Covid19 has certainly changed our lives forever. There are many lessons that can be learnt.

Health

Covid19 has shown up the vulnerable in our society. Make no mistake, if the pandemic had taken hold in Australia as it did in some other countries like Italy, our governments would have acted in a similar way. People over 65 and with chronic conditions would have become expendable to make beds available in hospitals for younger people. Although governments will not acknowledge this, consider the New South Wales Government's early reluctance to transfer people from aged care facilities to hospitals despite relatives pleading for this to happen. The New South Wales Health Department was unsure how dire the situation may get and were keen to keep hospital beds and ventilators available in case the pandemic did spread quickly and out of control.

Thankfully, our doctors were not placed in the terrible position of choosing who could and could not go onto ventilators in intensive care units in our hospitals.

For those that have contracted Covid19, it is unknown at this stage what the full and long term effects of the virus might be and if they have built up immunity to the virus or to the mutations now being found (such as those commonly known as the UK strain, South African strain or the Brazil strain). As the months go by, it is evident that the virus affects people differently; some recover relatively quickly, others take many months or maybe years. Some recent advice is that the virus can affect all parts of the body – heart, lungs, brain, kidneys and liver. What the long term effects will be on the body and our health care system is unknown. An expert at the Fiorey Institute has predicted that as Covid19 can inflame the brain then there is a likelihood of a dramatic increase in the incidence of neurological diseases like Parkinson's occurring. This prediction is based on research following the Spanish Flu pandemic where there was a dramatic increase in Parkinson's disease five years after the pandemic.

During the first six months of Covid19, we saw a dramatic increase in the use of telehealth – phone and video meetings with doctors and specialists. People were reluctant to leave their house for fear of catching the virus. Doctors became increasingly concerned that, with people not having regular check-ups with their doctors, cancers, diabetes and other diseases would go undetected in their early stages. It appears that telehealth is here to stay and, consequently, some specialists are predicting an increase in cases of cancers and other diseases that have gone undiagnosed during our first year with Covid19.

Scientists around the world were working on fast tracking a vaccine for the virus. Some were still in the final phases of trials before they became available and released for use in Britain and the USA. Russia has claimed to have a vaccine but it appears that some clinical trials have been bypassed in order to be the first. There are now a number of vaccines available but there is no understanding of how long a vaccine may last. Some of the vaccines like the Pfizer vaccine require that they be kept very cold (-70C) which will have implications in terms of transportation and availability. The vaccine being developed by the University of Queensland had the advantage of only requiring refrigeration but, unfortunately, it produced false positives for HIV during trials and has been discontinued.

One of the most unfortunate phrases to be used extensively during Covid19 was social distancing. The correct terminology should have been physical distancing; maintaining 1.5 metres between you and other people. Social distancing is not something that we require during this time. The Commonwealth Government has committed millions of dollars to addressing mental health and domestic violence caused by the lockdowns and loss of employment as a result of combatting the virus. It is more important than ever to maintain our social contacts, not to 'social distance'.

When we were in lockdown in Brisbane, we made it a point every couple of weeks to have a meetup with our gym buddies via Skype for a coffee or a wine. Once the restrictions were lifted, we again started having coffees together in our regular coffee shop, keeping our physical distance as required at the time.

In an earlier chapter, we discussed the importance of building and maintaining friendships and Covid19 has highlighted the importance of this. We have seen random acts of kindness where neighbours or even complete strangers have helped others who couldn't go shopping, others have had their lawns mowed and for others it was simply a matter of being contacted to make sure they were alright.

We have also seen people encouraging others to maintain their sense of humour by dressing up and occasionally dressing down to put the rubbish bins on the kerbside for collection.

Our national pride continued. Anzac Day marches, commemorative services and public gatherings were cancelled but people, street after street, instead remembered our fallen by joining their neighbours on their driveways and footpaths with their candles, torches and radios. In our neighbourhood, we could hear two buglers sound the last post.

Major sporting events like the grand finals of the Rugby League and AFL were held.

Physical exercise

With gyms closed as a result of the virus, more people started riding, jogging and walking. Families were exercising together, particularly walking and riding. There was an increase in bicycle and gym equipment sales. Unfortunately, in our area, the number of helmets didn't appear to match the number of bicycle sales so there was an increase in the number of people riding without helmets.

There was an increase in exercise videos being shown on various media outlets. Early in the pandemic, weights and other exercise equipment sold out in most stores. A few innovative people that I know found ways to make their own weights for example using two plastic milk bottles and sand. Once the restrictions were lifted, people could go back to gyms, often to restricted attendance. Initially, our gym restricted classes to six participants, the floor area was divided into six squares and it was within that area that exercises were undertaken. At the end of a session, the equipment used was sanitised. It was good to get back to gym sessions.

Twelve months after the first Covid19 case in Australia, much of the exercise equipment that had sold in the early days of Covid19 is now being sold through Ebay or similar as people are able to go back to the gym and no longer use their equipment at home.

Travel

For one who likes to travel, the period of self-isolation at home has been difficult. We would hear the occasional plane overhead but we had no plans to travel. Early in 2020, we had booked a number of flights and one-by-one these flights were cancelled resulting in a credit for future travel or a refund that seemed to take forever to be credited to our credit card.

Like many people, we took to looking at photos of past trips or identifying and researching countries to visit when opportunities to travel arose.

It didn't take too long before travel restrictions were applied both internationally and domestically. New South Wales, Victoria and the Australian Capital Territory were the only states and territory that did not initially close their borders. With other states and territories, travel was severely restricted. Even within states, in the early stages of Covid19 and again at other times following a potential outbreak, there were restrictions on how far one could travel from home.

Many Grey Nomads were caught out by Covid19. Many became homeless as states closed their borders and they found it difficult to find a place to park their caravan etc. Police checked caravan parks allowing only permanent residents to stay. Many that would normally have headed north during the winter months found they were ill-prepared for the winter in the southern states.

We were fortunate to be able to travel to the Northern Territory and during this trip spoke to a number of Grey Nomads and some not so grey. Many, particularly those from Western Australia, mentioned having been on the road for months and unable to return home due to border closures. The most common reason for wanting to return home was to see their grandchildren.

Even when international travel for Australians was banned and Australia closed its borders to international visitors, Australia was still allowing relief flights carrying stranded Australians returning from many parts of the world. A few months later, states placed limits on the numbers of returning travellers that they would accept each week. It took some time before these limits were increased.

Cases of the UK and South African strain of the virus reaching Australia resulted in Australia again reducing the number of passengers per week that states would accept. This caused frustration and anger for Australians overseas trying to return home. This was compounded by some airlines like Emirates cancelling flights to Australia and then later the UK government refusing flights to and from the United Arab Emirates.

While the Australian government has increased the number of repatriation flights, they have also increased some requirements, for example, passengers requiring Covid19 testing and a negative result within three days of flying home. These Covid19 tests are expensive and unfortunately there is never any guarantee that the flight may not be cancelled. There have also been reports of some airlines only selling business and first class seats on flights to Australia. One wonders whether a person with status (gold or platinum) with an airline would have a better chance of securing seats and whether these could be purchased using points.

Around the world, we saw a number of airlines file for bankruptcy or go into provisional liquidation or administration, Virgin Australia being the Australian example of one of the airlines being grounded. Airlines around the world mothballed aircraft despite the many thousands of dollars per week in maintenance costs even for grounded aircraft. Many airlines are seriously examining their fleets. Large bodied aircraft like the Boeing 747 and the A380 are unlikely to return to the skies for many airlines.

International travel is unlikely to return until 2022 at the earliest although there may be travel bubbles like between Australia and New Zealand and maybe to the Pacific Islands. Already travel companies are offering deals to Europe, South Pacific and the USA with discounts and flexibility.

With international flying cancelled and domestic flying severely restricted, airlines around the world extended frequent flyer memberships and status through until 2021 and some airlines through to 2022.

International flights for most Australians are unlikely before 2022. Masks at airports and on flights are now mandatory and likely to be a travel requirement for some time to come. The CEO of QANTAS, Mr Alan Joyce, is seeking to have it mandatory for passengers on QANTAS international flights to have been vaccinated and provide documentary evidence. The proposal is for a vaccine certificate similar to that for Yellow Fever vaccinations.

As vaccines start to roll out and people are vaccinated, a number of airlines are now contemplating a requirement for all passengers to be vaccinated.

Many of the hotel chains also extended their membership renewals. A number of the hotels and airlines also had very attractive offers to encourage members to buy credits for future travel and hotel stays. Hilton Hotels and Alaskan Airlines had very attractive offers during this period.

We had just returned from a Pacific Island cruise in January 2020, just a few weeks before things became serious, and met many who love cruising. We met many people that were on their sixth, tenth or twentieth cruise. For many of them, they will start cruising again as soon as cruises are allowed. Unfortunately, cruising has not had a great record with numerous cruises reporting outbreaks of stomach bugs and this was long before the disaster of the Ruby Princess and other cruise liners around the world reported cases of Covid19.

On our cruise, one of the activities that we undertook involved a tour of the galley. It was not an extensive tour but it did give an insight into where meals were prepared and how they came to the dining table from the galley. One disturbing thing that we saw, and was noticed by others on the tour, was one of the kitchen staff preparing food without any gloves.

Some commentators are saying that Covid19 will signal the end of the buffet and perhaps the live shows that cruises are known for. On our cruise the buffet was certainly popular amongst the young people in particular as there was a far greater choice of food and greater hours that the food was available. It meant that a person could have vegetarian, roast, pizza or Indian curry meals and a dessert in a short period of time then participate in other activities even if it was lounging around the pool drinking. At peak times, seating in these areas was at a premium and, although staff would take used plates, trays and cutlery from the tables, there was little time to wipe the tables down. Eating in the restaurants was more formal with two sitting times, a reduced but good choice of food over three courses and all meals served by wait staff.

We were fortunate that we had a suite on our cruise so we had a balcony and could turn the air conditioning off once we settled in. Those with inside cabins or just a porthole are reliant on the air conditioning and unfortunately the air conditioning could aid the spread of any infections on board.

Cruising is a major industry worldwide and a multi-million dollar industry in Australia. The cruise ships that call various ports in Australia home during the cruise season are all ships registered in overseas ports. It will be interesting to see if the shipping lines can implement changes required to reduce the likelihood of infection amongst passengers and crew. It can be anticipated that various governments like Australia and New Zealand will enforce stricter requirements regardless of where ships are registered.

Overseas there have been cruises undertaken by smaller ships utilising various methods to combat Covid19 such as requiring negative tests before boarding the ship. Unfortunately, each cruise ended with Covid outbreaks resulting in shortened cruises and quarantining.

By Christmas 2020, the much awaited travel bubble between Australia and New Zealand had not yet eventuated although travellers are allowed into Australia from New Zealand but have to quarantine for 14 days on their return to New Zealand. For Australians to travel to New Zealand without quarantine it was anticipated in March 2021 but the Northern Beaches cluster in December 2020 further delayed this travel bubble. The Australian government is prohibiting travel out of Australia unless a person has a valid reason to do so.

Housing

Covid19 has seen some extremes in predictions of what may happen to the value of houses as a result of Covid19. We have seen commentators predicting a fall of 30 percent, the CBA predicting 32 percent and others promoting no better time than now to purchase property for example 'property prices predicted to surge by 15 percent by 2023'. Now, more than ever, there is confusion about what will happen to the housing market. Figures around mid-year showed falls of around 12 percent in Sydney and Melbourne and two percent in Brisbane residential property prices but by the end of the year the housing market was strong again. Remember, there is no one property market. Prices may fall in one city or region and be rising in other areas. Pre Covid, there had been reports of a major housing shortage. Will Covid19 reduce this housing shortage? Certainly, for the next few years at least, there will be minimal migration to Australia so that should lessen the need for housing and reduce rents. The residential rental market is also likely to see more vacancies and lower rents particularly those properties that had relied on students. The other segment of the residential market that had suffered was those properties used for short term rentals like Airbnb. At the beginning of the pandemic, many were taken off the Airbnb type market and placed onto the normal residential rental market seeking tenants for six or twelve months. With interstate borders now reopening, the Airbnb style rentals should start to see occupancy increase although unlikely up to previous levels as overseas tourists are still restricted from entering Australia. Unlike many hotels that have a policy now of refunding if a cancellation is a result of a lockdown, Airbnb has no such policy.

In January 2021, house prices in Brisbane and some other cities increased. Brisbane is becoming home to people from Sydney and Melbourne. As a result, the Brisbane property market for houses and rentals is very strong - a seller's market. House prices and rents have increased dramatically. Covid19 has also seen a move by people from cities to regional areas particularly if their work allows them to work from home for most of the week. Consequently, house prices in many regional areas are the strongest they have been for years.

Expats who have been living abroad are now returning in large numbers and require places to live. They have helped take up the surplus in the apartment markets. Those predicting the large drops in the housing market may not have factored in these expats returning to Australia and seeking housing. The expats are also said to be responsible for the increase in the price of second hand vehicles in Australia.

Australia is also experiencing major shortages or delays in building materials due to new buildings and renovations being undertaken.

Covid19 has certainly shown up a number of issues in aged care facilities. A Royal Commission had started before Covid19 and now has many more issues to investigate. On the surface, there appears to be some major failings of this system. The Federal Government provides funding but the states administer the facilities. There appears to be not only understaffing but an inappropriate mix of staff; some facilities reported not having any nurses on staff. Furthermore it appears that many staff worked at more than one facility which resulted in the virus spreading across facilities.

Why did New South Wales and Victoria have the death toll that they did compared with other states and territories? Before anyone goes into an aged facility they should consider things such as the staffing levels, the mix of staff and what rights relatives have to remove parents if such a virus was to enter the facility. In Victoria, most cases have occurred in privately-owned rather than state-run aged care homes. Is the profit motive more important than the welfare of the residents in these privately operated institutions? Is there a breakdown between these homes and the Commonwealth agencies that fund them and, if so, why not with the privately operated institutions in other states and territories?

Prior to the pandemic, less than 30 per cent of older Australians lived in aged care facilities. Are older people more likely to stay in their own homes longer as a result of Covid19? With regard to an outbreak of a virus like Covid19, some retirement homes have proven to be unsafe and the virus has quickly spread. Some older people, particularly with dementia, have chosen to stay in familiar surroundings such as their rooms rather than go to hospital and some have health directives not to be resuscitated. These are a few of the reasons given by aged care facilities for why some aged care residents were not moved to hospitals.

While it is hard on relatives, some governments like Queensland locked down aged care homes, prisons and hospitals when there was an outbreak in the community. This was to reduce any risk of the virus entering the facilities and spreading rapidly in these confined areas.

Apartments, in particular inner-city apartments, have been hit hard by Covid19 as both prices and rentals have fallen. In some cities, like Brisbane, there had already been an oversupply and this has worsened. Most capital cities still have a number of large apartment complexes still to be completed and there may be further distress for these purchasers when valuations come in below purchase price and lenders require the purchaser to commit more funds. The anticipated rental incomes are also likely to be less than expected and if purchasing using borrowed money, then the purchaser may need to commit further funds each month.

I was recently speaking to a gentleman who has a twenty-year-old son with an intellectual disability. Covid19 has certainly made him think about the future of his son. Over the years, he has seen people in their seventies and eighties concerned about what will happen to their disabled children who may now be in their forties or fifties. The gentleman that I was speaking to explained that police had been called to their home on three occasions when their son had episodes. He was also now scared for his wife's safety now that his son had grown up and was quite strong. He felt that the best solution for his son was to find a house that he could call home and maybe share the house with someone who also has a disability. It is not a quick solution with various hurdles such as finding a suitable house and a compatible person to share the house with plus ensuring that they have the skills required to live away from his parents. In the long term, it is a good solution. His parents can provide some support now but be confident that when they are no longer able to offer any care, or they have passed, their son will have a home and be able to live a productive life, earning an income and being able to live independently with some ongoing support from trained professionals.

Hobbies

With the initial restrictions and lockdown in parts of Australia, people have had to look to ways of occupying their time. It seems many people have turned to gardening, particularly growing their own vegetables. Visits to our local Bunnings store showed most vegetable punnets were sold out. A similar occurrence with sewing items as people had returned to sewing. My daughter-in-law undertook to make face masks and send them to friends in Victoria.

Other people have turned to doing 500 or 1000 piece puzzles to occupy their time. Hundreds of others have undertaken family history research. The University of Tasmania, for example, has an online diploma course on family history and people undertaking that course are finding out that it is much more than just names and dates. Exploring the background of relatives, where they lived, the economic and social conditions of the time, how many may have lived in the house at the time of a census or even their cause of death can be extremely interesting.

Many others have started new hobbies or returned to hobbies that they haven't looked at for some time due to work commitments. People have found that they need activities other than watching Netflix to keep their minds active.

Generally, the lockdowns have been tough on people. Hobbies are important for keeping the mind active and for social contact.

Financial aspect

The financial effects of Covid19 have been many and varied. We have all read and heard about the mass retrenchments, unemployment, underemployment, the Commonwealth Job Seeker and Job Keeper programs as well as various state and territory programs. Much of the focus has been on the young and particularly those in industries such as hospitality and the travel industries. There are many more industries and livelihoods that have been affected; for example the tertiary education sector. There are many people who may have been considering retiring in the next few years, now finding themselves without employment and little prospect of obtaining future work.

For retirees or those planning to retire, many rely on dividends and interest from banks and term deposits. During the last twelve months, these have fallen sharply and that has certainly affected the income of self-funded retirees. While there has been some relief for those on government pensions, there has been no such assistance for self-funded retirees. The other popular source of income for retirees has been from residential rental income and again, for many, this has also reduced with government policy going against landlords even if tenants are unable to pay any rent. The short term rental market has been severely hit, now relying on domestic travellers rather than overseas visitors. Frequent border closures by various state governments have seen many people now feeling safer to holiday in their own state rather than being forced to quarantine for fourteen days if there is an outbreak.

As previously mentioned, Australia, like most countries in the world, is now in recession. Adam Creighton, the Economic Editor for The Australian referred to the recession currently as the Phoney Recession and that the worst is yet to come once the likes of Job Keeper and Job Seeker are reduced. There is a big question mark over what will happen to the housing market and other areas once some of these government stimulus packages are rolled back or removed. Many employers, particularly in our agricultural sector, have spoken of not being able to obtain labourers because the stimulus packages do not encourage people to look for work.

I am old enough to remember past recessions, one where we had runs on our financial institutions resulting in some being forced to close and taken over by others. This is unlikely to happen in this pandemic and as shown in the Global Financial Crisis, the Australian Government backed the banks.

I am not downplaying the seriousness of the current situation; I was working for a finance company in 1974 when Australia entered a recession. The company retrenched staff first using a 'last on, first off' philosophy so, while not the first to go, eventually my turn came. Fortunately, I was not unemployed for too long but certainly remember my thoughts and concerns at the time.

Some areas of the economy have suffered more than others. Those associated with the travel industries including airlines, cruising, hotels or locals associated with reef/dive/charter boat/ bus tours are well known to have suffered as a result of Covid19. To a lesser degree is the effect that Covid19 has had on other industries such as education and, in particular, the tertiary sector. Overseas students are unlikely to be allowed back into Australia until at least towards the end of 2022. Overseas students are full-paying students and therefore an important source of funds for the universities. Universities across Australia have had to seek voluntary redundancies of staff and cutback on research. In late November 2020, about sixty-three students from China, Vietnam,

Hong Kong, Japan and Indonesia arrived in Darwin to resume their study. Some other universities have proposed bringing students in from overseas but to date the hurdles for achieving this appear too great.

Recent information released shows that Australia has returned to about ninety per cent of pre- Covid19 employment levels although not in similar fields of employment.

Early in the pandemic we saw a number of Australian companies quickly adapt to making needed supplies like hand sanitisers and ventilators. The pandemic highlighted a need for Australia to have a manufacturing base that could adapt to producing critical supplies and for there to be adequate storage for a minimal level of these supplies so that we were not reliant on overseas supplies. The pandemic has provided our government with an opportunity to identify nationally what are critical infrastructure, goods and services that we need to have the capabilities of producing in Australia to be self-reliant.

Unfortunately, our memories of shortages in critical areas including pharmaceuticals will fade as we return to a new normal.

Unfortunately Covid19 and the recession highlight the need for people approaching retirement to be prepared a few years before their planned retirement date. Events do happen unexpectedly whether that is through redundancy, ill-health or a pandemic.

The economic climate that we are in with the recession, low interest rates and low inflation means that we need to look at our personal budget. Whatever our income source, we need to look at a worst-case scenario and be realistic. Our income is unlikely to improve during the recession so we need to control our expenses. Let's look at discretionary and non-discretionary spending; are there any areas that can be cut back or even eliminated altogether?

If you have a negatively-geared or slightly positive cashflow residential property, should you retain or sell? Each state and territory has had a moratorium on evicting tenants and tenants have received rent reductions if they have lost their jobs or had their hours reduced so landlords have been hurting even in times of very low interest rates. The Prime Minister's 'sympathetic' gesture has been problematic for many landlords. One writer has described this as 'a Robin Hood style attempt to steal from the rich landlord Peter to feed poor tenant Paul'. Politicians fail to understand that most landlords are not rich. Most own just one rental property and generally have a mortgage and claim negative gearing through the tax system. For those in retirement relying on the rental income to live on, this has been a body blow when they are already suffering from poor dividends and low returns from term deposits and bank interest due to Covid19.

Banks have offered repayment holidays but this is only a temporary relief and interest on any borrowings is still accruing. Governments have been talking of a housing-led recovery by building new housing but what is that likely to do for existing housing? One of the major contributors of housing demand has been migration but this has 'stopped'. There is an oversupply of apartments so that is also likely to put downward pressure on rents in some areas. The offset for many years of the poor yield from residential property has been the capital growth that people could expect but with low inflation and lack of demand, that capital growth may be hard to achieve in the next few years.

The Australian Government allowed workers affected by Covid19 to access up to $20,000 from their superannuation in two instalments over two financial years. Long term, this will be detrimental to those who have accessed their superannuation as they will miss the compounding effect over the years. Recent figures have shown that on average about $7,400 has been withdrawn. Over the year there have also been reports of superannuation withdrawals to fund purchases such as cars. Whether the Australian Taxation Office will investigate everyone that has withdrawn funds from their superannuation during this period is not yet known and if they do, and a breach is found, will there be any penalties applied?

The Commonwealth Government had been hoping that the Job Seeker and Job Keeper payments may have stimulated the economy by people spending but people fearful of the future have been putting money into their savings.

Commercial property investments do not appear to have been as affected by rent reductions. Many of the shops that closed are likely to have been on month-by-month tenancies. Some larger companies like Flight Centre and some large clothing chains have seen the closure of some stores as a result of Covid19. Business owners generally take their legal obligations of a lease seriously and it is important for them to have premises to operate from. In many areas, the yield in commercial properties has decreased as more people look for property with long leases and better returns.

We have seen stories of many scams occurring during Covid19, relying on people's generosity to help the less fortunate but ultimately only lining the pockets of con artists Many of these con artists prey on the elderly so it is wise to have a strategy in place and stick to that plan. If you wish to deviate then ask some other trusted people and do some research before committing any funds.

There have been some promoters extolling the virtue of Bitcoin, gold and silver a few months after the pandemic started. Gold has traditionally been a commodity that people have purchased during times of crisis like wars and economic uncertainty. Now, people are promoting Bitcoin as better than gold. It has certainly increased in value in recent months, now selling for around $40,000 per Bitcoin in Australia. It is claimed that Bitcoin is now maturing into a hedge against inflation similar to gold and is no longer seen as a form of universal currency. It is claimed that many institutional investors like hedge funds and banks are now buying Bitcoin unlike in the 2017 Bitcoin boom when it was retail investors. This would suggest Bitcoin is now out of the reach for retail investors and many will now look at other cryptocurrencies hoping it may replicate Bitcoin. Recently Elon Musk, currently the world's richest man, announced a major purchase of Bitcoin and possible use of Bitcoin to purchase Tesla vehicles. One has to wonder about the motive of such a public announcement that pushed the price of Bitcoin to around US$48,000. We have seen Bitcoin again drop in price. Will we see a dramatic drop in the price again as we have in the past? History would suggest that we will and those who have bought at or near the top of the price surge will suffer a substantial loss. Amazon is one company reportedly developing its own cryptocurrency. If Amazon and a few other large companies develop their own cryptocurrency, what will happen to the price of Bitcoin? If you are contemplating purchasing Bitcoin or any cryptocurrency, I would suggest buying our book *Blockchain, Cryptocurrencies & The Future* for an unbiased look at what is required to purchase and hold cryptocurrency and tax implications.

One promoter has recommended short term rentals as the next boom area for investors but using a more risky strategy of using other people's property. In times of uncertainty, stay away from risky strategies or the potential 'boom and bust get-rich-quick' schemes.

Whilst Australia is a very large island and could close its borders to secure the health of its population, that is never likely to happen. It has been estimated that there are over one million Australians travelling overseas during any year and the borders need to remain open to allow Australian citizens to return or, as is becoming more common with Covid19, to repatriate these travellers. Also our tourist industry relies heavily on overseas visitors. So, while theoretically Australia could close its borders, for various reasons this will never be the situation.

Social

The last year has been challenging in many ways. There have been lockdowns in various areas, restrictions on how many people can attend weddings, funerals, churches and gather in homes. It has been a very difficult year for those in aged care homes and hospitals; particularly if relatives live interstate. I know of a number of people who have parents in their 90s who haven't been able to visit them for over 12 months.

People have had to wait months to be able to see newborn grandchildren. At times, there have been restrictions on who can be present during the birth of a child and some fathers have not been allowed to be present. We have had hundreds of weddings, engagement parties and birthday parties cancelled or sometimes hurriedly brought forward due to restrictions on the number of people that can come together. It has been difficult during Covid19 to plan anything without a backup plan. Telephone calls and skype sessions do help but they can't replace face-to-face contact.

Our home lives have been disrupted with requirements to work from home and for our children to study at home. Parents have taken on roles as teachers even if only for supervision. Our children have missed the social interaction with their classmates and workers with their fellow workers.

Slowly things are starting to return to some normality with children back to school and people returning to their offices and factories.

Ongoing disruption to our social activities is likely to continue for some time as small outbreaks occur and until most of the population is vaccinated.

For many people, one of the positive outcomes of Covid19 has been people realising how important their social networks are. More than ever, we need to be maintaining and developing our social networks.

Reinventing yourself

Sadly, many people have lost their jobs as a result if Covid19. For a number, particularly in the 50 plus age bracket, the likelihood of gaining employment diminishes with age.

Have you considered what you may do if you were to lose your job with little likelihood of regaining employment? Would you look at starting a business or look to retrain in another field? There are government assisted programs for retraining available. It may not be retraining into a job; there are many organisations seeking people such as Meals on Wheels or Men's Shed. Reinventing yourself is not necessarily about money but more of connecting with people and maintaining a sense of purpose.

Even if you are forced to retire before you intended and are able to gain the pension, or have sufficient funds to provide for your retirement, what will you do with all your spare time? Covid19 has suddenly made thinking about reinventing yourself a reality for many middle-aged Australian workers.

A person I know retired a little over a year ago and is starting to reinvent himself in aged care. Money is not the objective here as he is comfortable financially and, after years of managerial positions, any supervisory or management role is certainly not wanted. It was more a matter of meeting other people and having a sense of being useful. There is a real need in this area and there may be government packages to cover the training costs.

Reinventing yourself does not necessarily mean finding other employment. It is really a matter of finding a new identity that you are happy with and people may associate you with. In many ways, it is not about how other people see you; it is what you are comfortable with. It could be volunteering at a charity, it could be fishing, bowls or golf or you may want to be president, secretary or treasurer of a club or body corporate. How you wish to reinvent yourself is a personal decision and, over your lifetime in retirement, it may change a number of times. Not having to do something for money, recognition or social status can be very rewarding.

Planning for the inevitable

Covid19 has also created a great deal of stress for many families; losing family members to the virus or other health issues. State and territory governments placed restrictions on how many people could attend funerals. At times state borders were closed and some governments even heartlessly refused applications on compassionate grounds to see dying relatives and stopped family members from interstate attending funerals unless they had undertaken 14 days quarantine.

A large funeral or even a viewing may not always be possible so, if planning your funeral, consider some options.

Covid19 has not discriminated in who it will infect and people from early 20s to 100 have died. The virus highlights the need to plan for the unexpected and the inevitable. Have you prepared your Will, Enduring Power of Attorney and Health Directives?

Final words

Australia has done well in containing the pandemic. Yes there are, and will be, the occasional outbreaks to form regional clusters but I am confident that each state and territory has the capability through their contract tracing and genomic sequencing to quickly bring these under control. Will the vaccine provide an end to Covid19? Unlikely, as we have seen the virus mutate and this is likely to continue. Scientists around the world did well to develop all these various vaccines but they can't rest on their laurels. All vaccines will need to be further developed to address these new mutations and maybe provide longer benefits.

Australia has not rushed into approval of any Covid19 vaccines. The Therapeutic Goods Authority (TGA) has now approved the Pfizer and the AstraZeneca vaccines for use in Australia. Australia also has contracts to purchase two other vaccines, Novavax and Moderna. Australia is also one of about 188 countries around the world to join Covax aiming to support fair and equitable access to Covid19 vaccines. It also enables Australia to purchase new vaccines as they become available.

While there are still some unknowns about the vaccines, such as how long they may provide protection and whether they will stop the transmission of the virus, the vaccines are an integral part of combatting the virus. Even one dose of the vaccine seems to lessen the severity of Covid19 resulting in less likelihood of hospitalisation.

Australia will not make vaccinations compulsory but there are some industries where voluntary vaccination may not be possible. It is likely that there will be some legal challenges regarding working conditions and vaccinations. It is unlikely that Australia's borders will reopen to the rest of the world until the majority of the Australian population is vaccinated. There are currently no indication of what percentage of the Australian population will be required to be vaccinated but it could be around 80 per cent of the adult population. Travel bubbles are likely in the interim to allow quarantine free travel between Australia and New Zealand, South Pacific islands and possibly Singapore.

It has been reported that, globally, it is likely to be around seven years to reach 75 per cent Covid19 immunity. Even at 75 per cent immunity, people may be reluctant to travel overseas and many will slowly and cautiously re-emerge into the post Covid19 world.

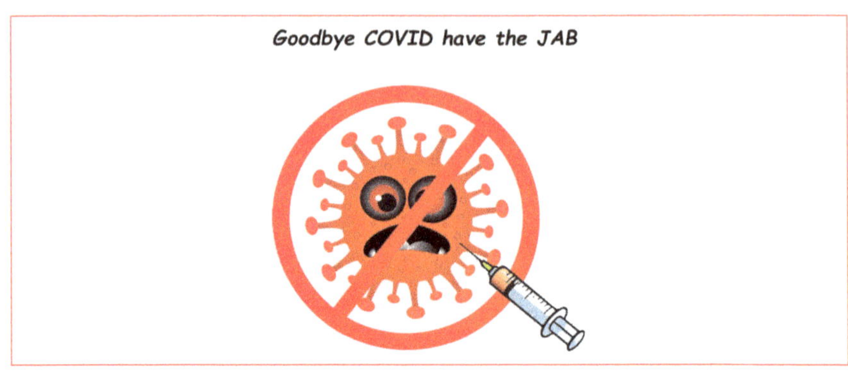

While Australia may have united to fight Covid19, each state and territory has taken a different view in the ways they protect their citizens. The hard, and sometimes swift, border closures that we have seen (for example in South Australia, Western Australia and greater Brisbane) are likely to continue as small outbreaks continue. It makes domestic travel, particularly interstate, very difficult to plan and one has to be prepared to cancel travel plans at short notice.

I am sure that, as it has for the last 12 months, the virus will continue to have outbreaks in Australia as more Australians attempt to come home. Over 200,000 residents have returned in the last 12 months and, despite an occasional breach, the hotel quarantine and strict border controls have worked well for Australia. The rollout of the vaccines should allow Australians greater freedom to travel within Australia, and hopefully the South Pacific, and to feel confident to undertake most things that they would like to do in retirement.

The final word, as it has been since the pandemic started, would have to be caution. It is likely to be a new world that we live in. We have to be prepared for changes. No longer can we plan for an interstate holiday and expect that we will be able to holiday as planned. How and where we work, and where we study may change. Our investments may change; low interest rates mean that living off bank interest and dividends may need to be reconsidered. Capital gains to offset poor rental yields are likely to be a thing of the past unless one is prepared to manufacture growth in residential properties.

In recent months, we have seen a group of small investors manipulate the share price of a company called Gamestop and the price of Bitcoin may also be included as one that has recently been manipulated. Be very cautious in following investments that are on massive rises.

We are in for some challenging but exciting times. As baby boomers, we are accustomed to changes and exciting times but with maybe fewer years ahead of us in which to recover from financial, health or social stress, be cautious but not afraid.

Key learnings from this chapter

Commercial Property Buyers Agency

As we have suggested earlier in this book, it is important to consider taking some profits made through cryptocurrencies and invest them in some main stream investments. *Commercial Property Buyers Agency* is a boutique company specialising in the purchase of commercial property, on behalf of its clients. The company is very active in the commercial property real estate market and in regular contact with many commercial real estate agents.

We will, as a buyer's agent, always work in the best interest of the client, and always look to secure a property at the lowest possible price and best terms. We understand time and budget constraints and will work within those to secure a property at a price and terms favourable to the client.

Our aim is to purchase a commercial property that meets our client's requirements, will attract and retain quality tenants, have good long-term leases and provide strong rental yield. Above all, we aim to save our clients time, money and stress. We are committed to always acting with integrity and honesty and in our client's best interest. If you would like to find out more about how *Commercial Property Buyers Agency* can find the right commercial property for you, or more about mentoring, contact cpbuyersagency@gmail.com. Visit our website www.cpbuyersagency.com.au

Other Books by the Authors

We hope that you have found the information in this book useful. If you have any questions, or if you would like to provide a testimonial, please email us at arthurphillipbooks@gmail.com.

Arthur Phillip Books is publishing six books in the next 12 months under the series title, *"It's My Time"*.

A key to success is to continually improve your financial competence and this series of books is designed to assist with improving your competency in property investment.

The first book in this series is titled *'It's My Time: The A to Z of Property and Financial Terms'*. It was designed as a resource, a useful reference for terminology, providing reference websites and some basic forms. It is designed to complement our next books in the series.

The second book titled *'It's My Time: Setting Financial and Personal Goals'* is about planning and developing a blueprint for the rest of your life, regardless of your age. Most people have no financial plan, nor a belief that they can be financially free. Many invest in shares and/or property with little thought as to why they are doing so, or how it will fit into their current or future, lifestyle.

The third book in the series is titled *'It's My Time: Successful Residential Investing'* then builds upon the first two and focusses on residential property investment. We will delve into aspects of being a landlord that aren't included in most books, for example abandoned goods and meth labs.

The fourth book titled *'It's My Time: Introducing Commercial Investing'* is about commercial real estate. Commercial real estate in the last couple of years has seen an increase in popularity as the yield from residential property declines. Many SMSFs are also looking at commercial property because of the returns and the long-term leases.

This book *'It's My Time: Planning a Holistic Retirement'* is the fifth book in this series. This book covers planning for retirement: not only financially but also how to transition from work life to retirement – where you may live, friendships outside of work, and what you will do to fill in your day without going to work: travel, volunteering, part time work, etc.

'It's My Time: Strategies in Action' is the sixth book in this series. This book is about planning and developing a blueprint for the rest of your life, regardless of your age. It is about taking what you have learnt in the other books and creating a strategy. One of the important things with establishing your strategy is that you follow your strategy, and repeat it, and keep repeating it. This is the secret to financial success: becoming a master at those things that make up your strategy and staying focused.

Blockchain, Cryptocurrencies & The Future is another book published by Arthur Phillip Book Publishing. This book will help you to understand the new and emerging world of blockchain and cryptocurrencies from an Australian layman's perspective. There is a common belief in the public that cryptocurrency is 'everything one does not understand about money combined with everything one does not understand about computers'. This book covers a wide range of topics including the history of money, cryptography, the origin and purpose of blockchain, the origin and purpose of digital currency, current uses and potential application, blockchain and its rivals, Australian taxation, purchasing goods and services, mining and trading, hacking and scams, how countries view cryptocurrencies, how banks are reacting (is it a bubble ?) and, finally, closing thoughts from the authors.

All pre-ordered books or additional copies purchased through our website receive a 10% discount off the listed price. If you would like to pre-order any of these books, visit our website www.arthurphillipbooks.com or email us at arthurphillipbooks@gmail.com. or contact us on +61-451-902-123.

Bibliography

Abey, Arun, and Andrew Ford. *How Much is Enough?: Making Financial Decisions that Create Wealth and Well-being*. Greenleaf Book Group, 2009.

Abey, Arun, and Andrew Ford. *How Much is Enough?* A & B Publishers, 2007.

Anthony, Mitch. *AARP The New Retirementality: Planning Your Life and Living Your Dreams... at Any Age You Want*. John Wiley & Sons, 2011.

Bernstein, Alan, and John Trauth. *Your retirement, your way: why it takes more than money to live your dream*. McGraw Hill Professional, 2006.

David Bogan and Keith Davies. *Avoid Retirement and Stay Alive: Why You Should Never Retire and How Not To*. HarperCollins Publishers (New Zealand) Limited, 2007

Buttrose Will, Buttrose Ita, Galgut Mike. *How much is Enough*. Lime Grove House Publishing, 2003.

Healey, Kaye. *Changing Course How Do I Retire*, Choice Books, 2002.

Hull, Alan. *Active Retirement*, Wrightbooks, 2005.

Longhurst, Michael. *The Beginner's Guide to Retirement–Take Control of Your Future: 6 Steps to a Successful and Stress-Free Retirement*. Gill & Macmillan Ltd, 2001.

Longhurst, Michael. *Enjoying Retirement*, Hachette Australia, 2018.

Manners. Bruce. *Retirement Ready*, Signs Publishing, 2016

Newnham, Max. *Funding Your Retirement*, Wrightbooks, 2011

Scandlyn, Joy. *Retire Right,* New Holland Publishers, 2007.

Scully, Paul. *Investing for your Retirement*, Information Australia, 1999.

Sheard, Robert. *Money for life: The 20 factor plan for accumulating wealth while you're young.* HarperBusiness, 2000.

Stein, Ben, and Phil DeMuth. *Yes, You Can Still Retire Comfortably!.* Hay House, Inc, 2006.

Tan, Philomena. *Leaving the rat race to get a life: A map for charting your sea change.* Wrightbooks, 2004.

Upton, David. *Rethink, Relax, Retire,* Pan McMillian, 2002

Yates, Cynthia. *Living well in Retirement*, Harvest House Publishers 2005.

Yogev, Sara. *A Couple's Guide to Happy Retirement,* Familus, 2012.